The Complete Book of
RELAXATION TECHNIQUES

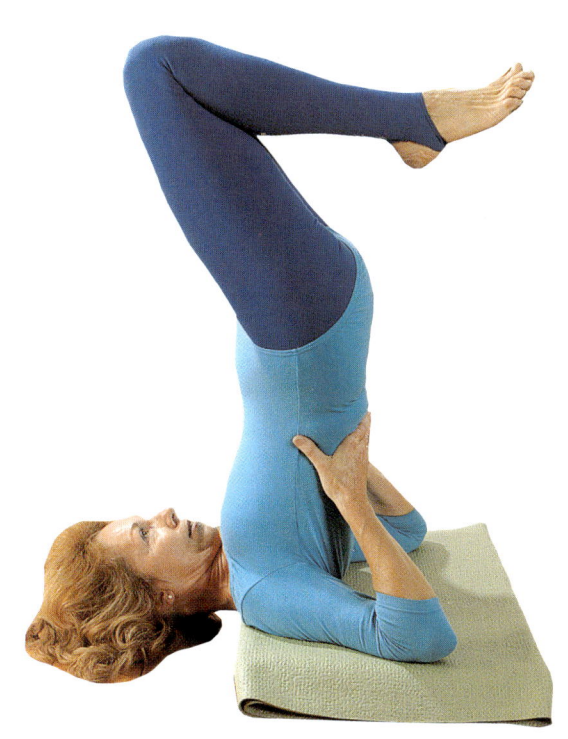

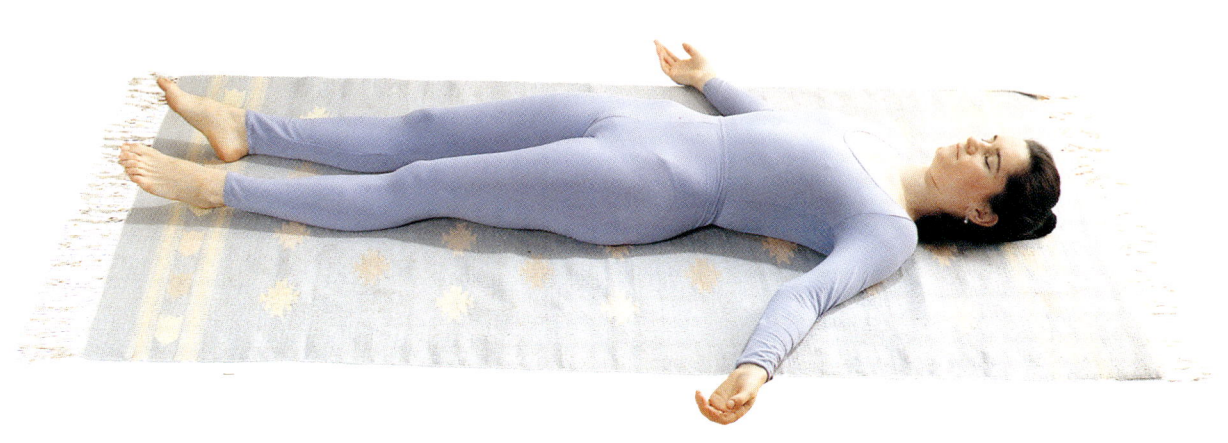
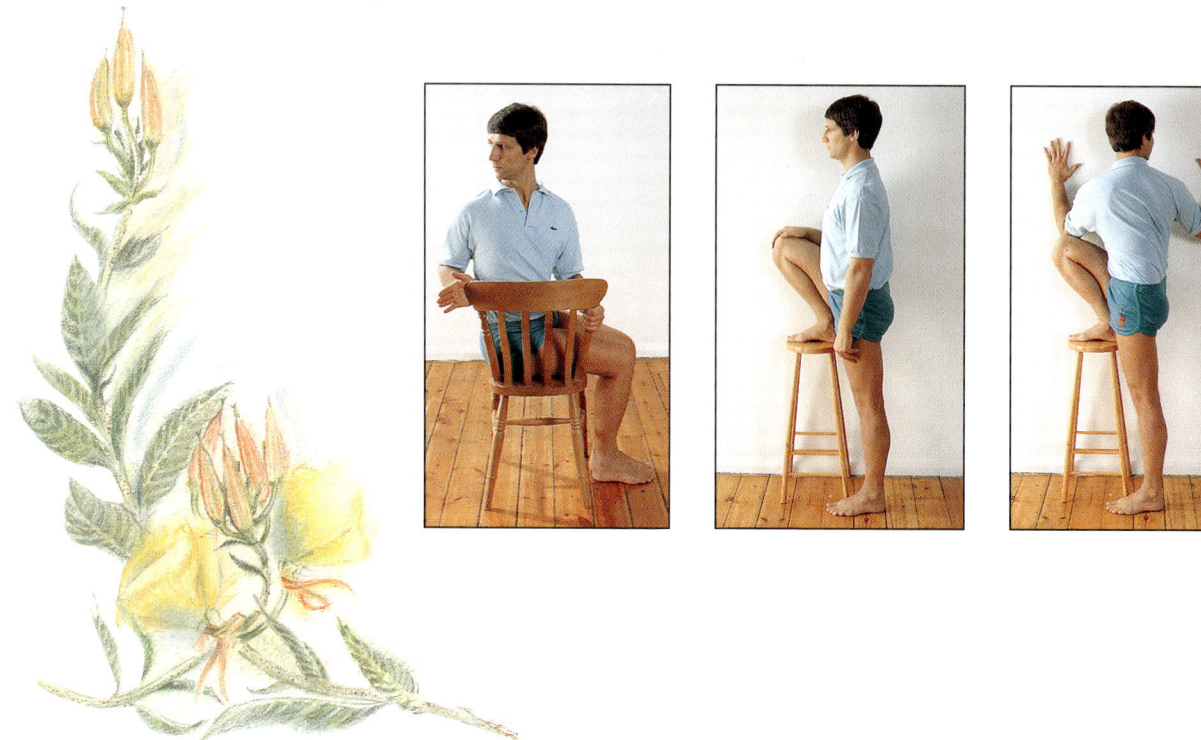

The Complete Book of
RELAXATION
TECHNIQUES

Develop your own anti-stress programme

from over 30 techniques – each one

illustrated and explained

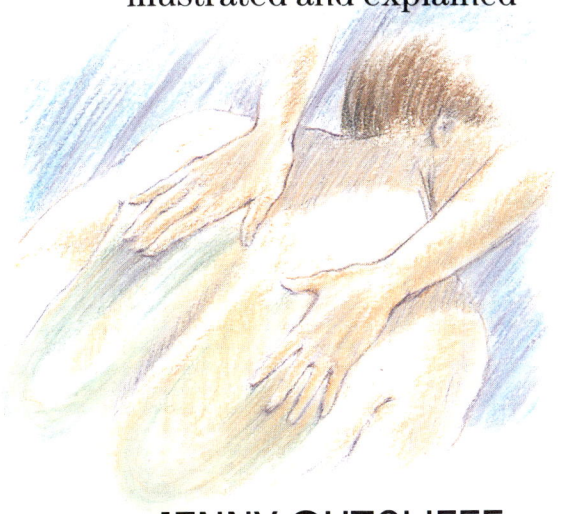

JENNY SUTCLIFFE

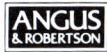

An imprint of HarperCollins*Publishers*

AN ANGUS & ROBERTSON BOOK

An imprint of HarperCollins Publishers

First published in Australia in 1991 by
CollinsAngus & Robertson Publishers Pty Limited (ACN 009 913 517)
A division of HarperCollins Publishers (Australia) Pty Limited
4 Eden Park, 31 Waterloo Road, North Ryde, NSW 2113, Australia

Copyright © 1991 Quarto Publishing plc

This book is copyright.
Apart from any fair dealing for the purposes of private study,
research, criticism or review, as permitted under the Copyright Act,
no part may be reproduced by any process without written permission.
Inquiries should be addressed to the publisher.

This book was designed and produced by
Quarto Publishing plc
6 Blundell Street
London N7 9BH

Senior Editor: Caroline Beattie
Editor: Candace Burch
Contributing Editor: Susan Berry
Designer: Hugh Schermuly
Photographer: Paul Forrester
Illustrator: Sharon Smith
Art Director: Nick Buzzard
Publishing Director: Janet Slingsby

National Library of Australia
Cataloguing-in-Publication data:
Sutcliffe, Jenny,
   The complete book of relaxation techniques
   ISBN 0207 17361 3.
     1. Relaxation. 2. Stress management. 1. Title.
613.79

Typeset by Bookworm Typesetting, Manchester
Manufactured in Hong Kong by Excel Graphic Arts Limited
Printed in Hong Kong by Leefung-Asco Printers Limited

4 3 2 1
95 94 93 92 91

CONTENTS

STRESS AND RELAXATION

Why do we Need to Relax?	8
Assessing your Stress	10
Relaxation Techniques	14
Personal Programmes	15
The Twenties	16
The Thirties	20
The Forties	24
The Fifties	28
The Sixties	32

SYMPTOM AND THERAPY FLOWCHARTS

Aches & Pains	38
Digestive Problems	40
Palpitations	42
Worry & Fuss	44
Insomnia & Fatigue	46
Hidden Problems	48
Anger	50
Depression	52

BASIC RELAXATION TECHNIQUES

Basic Relaxation Technique	56
Breathing Techniques	60
Posture	64
Warming-up and Stretching Exercises	66

RELAXATION TECHNIQUES

Massage	72
Aromatherapy	80
Smell Therapy	82
Acupressure/Do-in/Shiatsu	84
Reflexology	86
Metamorphic Therapy	89
Hydrotherapy	90
Floatation Tank	92
Negative Ion or Air Ionization Therapy	94
TENS Therapy	96
Sound Therapy	97
T'ai Chi Chuan	98
Yin and Yang	101
The Alexander Technique	102
The Feldenkrais Method	108
Yoga	110
Meditation	118
Autosuggestion/Couéism	120
Autogenic Therapy	121
Visualization Therapy	122
Self-Healing	124
Self-Hypnosis/Hypnotherapy	126
Biofeedback	129
Nutritional Medicine	130
Naturopathy	134
Herbalism	136
Evening Primrose Oil	137
Homoeopathy	138
Bach Flower Remedies	141
Colour Therapy	142
Chakras	145
Crystal and Gem Therapy	146
Dance Therapy and Eurhythmy	147
Music Therapy	148
Art Therapy	150
Pattern and Pyramid Therapy	152
Bibliography	154
Index	156
Credits	159

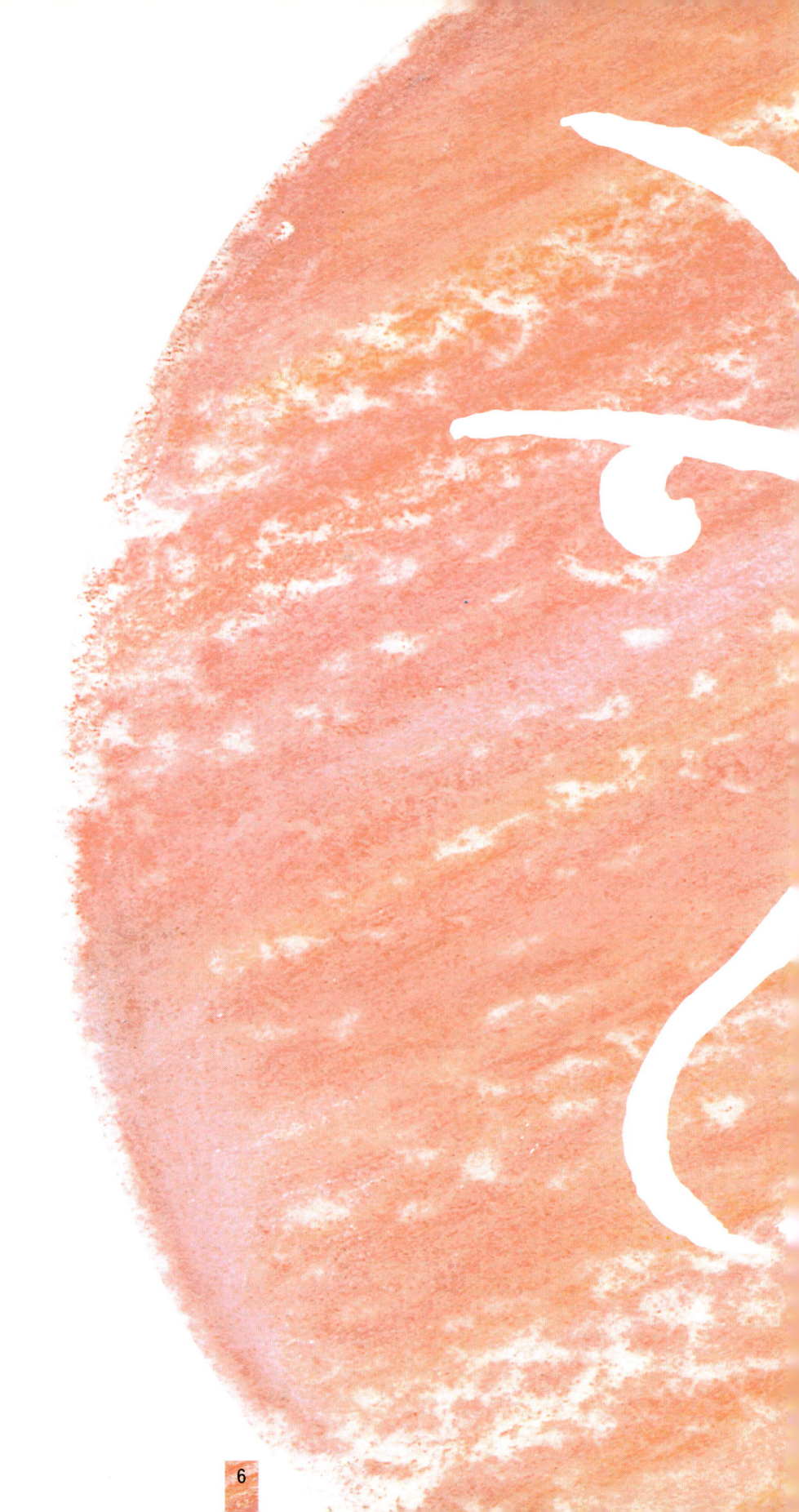

STRESS AND RELAXATION

The main benefit of relaxation is, paradoxically, a negative one: when you are relaxed, you are not stressed. (Of course, there are certain times when the stress response is necessary – it is prolonged, or long-term stress that is harmful). Even though true relaxation is rare in the modern world, in an ideal society it would be the normal condition of human beings – one in which contentment and lack of worry allows one to feel well, work well and be full of energy during the day; to sleep deeply at night; to deal with every situation calmly and competently; to form and sustain relationships with others; and to avoid undue stress.

Our world, of course, is far from relaxed and is full of stress. But that is no reason why we should not protect ourselves from bad stress and reduce its effect on our bodies and minds by relaxing using the techniques described in this book.

WHY DO WE NEED TO RELAX?

Stress and relaxation are opposite sides of the same coin, and both are necessary for a healthy life. When they are in balance all is well, but if stress predominates, illness often develops – the possible consequences can range from headaches, anxiety and lethargy through to heart attacks, ulcers or cancer. But while experts agree that stress plays a part in the onset and course of many disorders, it should be emphasized that not all stress is a bad thing. Even the best of times, like getting married, receiving a job promotion, going on holiday, or having a baby, are stressful, but good for you. All stress comes from two basic sources: physical activity and mental or emotional activity. Emotional frustration is more likely to cause stress-related disease, such as ulcers, than any type of physical work, though overwork accompanied by failure or lack of purpose can lead to exhaustion and even breakdown. However, the absence of work is no cure, and being excessively relaxed and indifferent to stress would mean missing out on all the wonderful feelings that add spice to life: euphoria, for example; excitement; heightened awareness of sounds, colour, and smells; exhilaration; a sense of triumphing over the odds; and the heady scent of success. A well-adjusted approach to life's inherent pressures implies the juggling of all kinds of stress – both positive and negative – in order to achieve the balance we strive for.

The physical response to the stress of a real or imagined threat is as old as human existence – and it is this very instinctive response that creates the problem. The 'fight or flight' response, as it is known, was well suited to our ancestors; unfortunately, nowadays many of the things that trigger our stress reactions do not require this response. We cannot run out of a meeting that we feel is going badly, or punch the chairman in the nose – if, that is, we wish to keep our jobs. We cannot run from a traffic jam or a supermarket queue, unless we are willing to lose the car and the groceries.

The word 'stress' is taken from engineering jargon; in essence it means the deformation or change caused on a body by the internal forces that work on it. The maximum stress a body can withstand and still return to its normal state is known as its 'elastic limit'. This applies to people, too: an individual has his or her own elastic limit, both in terms of degree and type of stress. It is when the body is put under long-term stress that it can reach its snapping point; if it does the damage can be irreparable.

The stress response – 'fight or flight' – breaks down, in physiological terms, into three stages:-

1 **Ready** – the threat is appreciated and the brain evaluates all the relevant information; the initial information is amplified through an instantaneous heightening of the senses. The whole process takes fractions of a second.

2 **Steady** – the body prepares for action, and chemical messengers, called hormones, are released by the brain to flood through the body, carried by the bloodstream. At the same time electrical impulses are fired through the nervous systems directly to the appropriate parts of the body. There are two types of nervous system:-

The voluntary, conscious system that is under our mental control – when, for example, we put out a hand to pick something up.

The involuntary, or autonomic system. This system controls the body without the need for conscious thought (though on occasion it can be influenced by conscious thought) 24 hours a day. It controls the body's vital organs and maintains a balance between their various functions. The autonomic system consists of two parts:-

The sympathetic system, which mainly controls the stress response and has a similar effect to the hormone system described below.

STRESS AND RELAXATION

The parasympathetic system, which deals mainly with the digestion, fights off infection, controls the immune response and tries to conserve energy. For example, during starvation – or excessive dieting – the parasympathetic system lessens the body's requirement for food, so that it can survive for longer. This also means that at the end of a diet the body's requirement for food is lowered and the parasympathetic system will greedily grasp all the food products that are available and store them as fat.

▪ The hormones, released in *Steady*, trigger the production of further hormones by two areas of the mid-brain (a primitive part of the brain) called the hypothalamus and the pituitary gland. These messengers, in their turn, stimulate the release of further hormones in other glands, such as the adrenal glands above the kidneys.

Adrenalin (also called epinephrine in America), produced by the adrenal glands, increases the heartbeat, raises the blood pressure, increases the rate of breathing and increases the sugar in the blood – this energy source is diverted to the muscles.

Endorphins, the body's own pain-relieving chemicals, which are produced in the brain, inhibit the appreciation of pain and give a feeling of euphoria.

Cortisol, also from the adrenal glands, increases the rate at which blood clots, and supplies energy to the vital organs by releasing stored fat in the form of glucose.

3 Go – both the actions of the sympathetic nervous system and the release of hormones have the effect of immediately increasing the level of oxygen in the lungs and the speed and efficiency with which this is transferred to the muscles. In addition, glucose stored in the body (in the form of glycogen) is released to give extra energy-power to the muscles.

▪ The parasympathetic system reduces its activity and diverts some of the supply of blood and nutrients from the internal organs, to augment the supply to the heart, lungs and muscles.

▪ The brain switches to a 'super-charged' state, with all the senses acute and alert to every nuance of vision, smell, hearing and atmosphere.

What we have just described is the body's response to a 'full alert'. Generally, though, we do not go past 'ready' and rarely in modern life do we need to reach 'go', except when taking exercise. This is why we suffer from so many symptoms of stress. The body is continually being prepared for 'fight or flight', but then has nowhere to go: modern, civilized modes of behaviour do not allow us to go on to the next stage. The body can dissipate a certain amount of the response, but when the stimulus is prolonged or excessive, and when there is no response, the ability to dissipate it fails, and the mechanism of the response ends up by attacking the body that it is trying to protect. The attack results in tension, stress, a lack of relaxation and a variety of signs and symptoms, some of which can have serious effects in the long term.

For our purposes, it does not matter whether the threat to which the body is responding is real or imaginary, since a threat that is purely in the mind is just as real, as far as the body is concerned, as one that is tangible, physical and close. Equally, people who kid themselves that there is no threat, or, at least, that they can cope with any threat that does exist, when in reality they cannot, will still suffer from stress symptoms as well. These two aspects of the problem often tend to set up a vicious circle, in which minor stresses create worry and uncertainty, which then become major threats, which in turn cause major stress – and so on.

ASSESSING YOUR STRESS

At some time in your life there will be some incident or event that causes major stress and may alter your lifestyle. Such crises are often known as life events. After interviewing thousands of people, researchers in America compiled a list of the most common life events that produced stress – not necessarily harmful stress – and devised a system of points for each event; the events include such emotional traumas as divorce, bereavement and moving house. The researchers discovered that our adaptability and ability to relax and cope with stress was damaged, often resulting in illness, if a person scored too many points in any one year.

100 points
a 10% increase in the risk
of illness over the next 2 years.
100–300 points
a 50% increase in the risk of
illness over the next 2 years.
300 & over
a dangerous risk of illness
over the next 2 years.

Everyone reacts differently to stress: some people naturally find one particular life event more damaging than another; and heredity, lifestyle and diet all affect an individual's response. Use this list as an initial reference, and add to it any other life events that you personally find stressful. Work out your own score by combining the two.

STRESS POINTS

Event	Points
Death of partner	100
Divorce	73
Separation from partner	65
Prison sentence	63
Death of close family member	63
Injury or illness to yourself	53
Marriage – your own	50
Given the sack at work	47
Reconciliation with partner	45
Retirement	45
Ill health in member of family	44
Pregnancy – your own	40
Sexual problems/difficulties	39
Addition of new family member	39
Major business or work changes	39
Change in your financial state	38
Death of friend	37
Change to a different type of work	36
More arguments with partner	35
Take on a large mortgage	31
Mortgage or loan foreclosed	30
Change in responsibilities at work	29
Child leaves home	29
Trouble with in-laws	29
Outstanding personal achievement	28
Wife begins or stops work	26
Child begins or ends school	26
Change in living conditions	25
Change of personal habits	24
Trouble with boss or employer	23
Change in working hours or conditions	20
Change in residence	20
Child changes schools	20
Change in church activities	19
Change in social activities	18
Change in sleeping habits	16
Change in number of family get-togethers	15
Change in eating habits	15
Holiday	13
Christmas (coming soon)	12
Minor violations of the law	11

The scale is adapted from Holmes and Rahe's Life Change Index; Journal of Psychosomatic Research, 1967, Vol. 11, pp. 213–218.

STRESS AND RELAXATION

SIGNS AND SYMPTOMS

Many common complaints and conditions can be the result of stress. But when one or more of the signs or symptoms below occur more frequently than normal, or are more difficult to shrug off, this can be an indication that your stress level is becoming unacceptably high.

Complete the quiz below, trying to be honest with your answers. If you tick four or more in the last box, and/or eight or more in the middle boxes, your stress level is unacceptably high. That means it is time to review your lifestyle and take steps to reduce stress.

EMOTIONAL SYMPTOMS

	RARELY	SOMETIMES	OFTEN
irritability and/or over excitability	☐	☐	☐
feeling depressed	☐	☐	☐
intolerance of others and/or yourself	☐	☐	☐
aggressiveness and/or anger	☐	☐	☐
suspiciousness	☐	☐	☐
fussiness – particularly over small things	☐	☐	☐
restlessness and/or impulsiveness	☐	☐	☐
tension and a feeling of being 'strung up'	☐	☐	☐
anxiety about small things	☐	☐	☐
despondency	☐	☐	☐
loss of concentration and/or memory	☐	☐	☐
feelings of frustration	☐	☐	☐
feelings of panic	☐	☐	☐
nightmares or disturbed dreams	☐	☐	☐
a feeling of being apart	☐	☐	☐
dithering about decisions	☐	☐	☐
frequent crying	☐	☐	☐
loss of interest in sex	☐	☐	☐
feeling of loss of control	☐	☐	☐
illogical worries and/or fears	☐	☐	☐

MEDICAL ALERT

If you are in any doubt about your health, visit your family doctor. Some of the signs and symptoms of stress can be similar to those produced by serious illnesses.

STRESS AND RELAXATION

BEHAVIOURAL SYMPTOMS

	RARELY	SOMETIMES	OFTEN
increased smoking	☐	☐	☐
increased alcohol consumption	☐	☐	☐
increased use of medication	☐	☐	☐
increased casual sex	☐	☐	☐
over-eating	☐	☐	☐
obsessive dieting or taking of laxatives	☐	☐	☐
gnashing or grinding of teeth	☐	☐	☐
an eye tic	☐	☐	☐
finger or foot tapping	☐	☐	☐
frowning	☐	☐	☐
nail-biting	☐	☐	☐
scratching the scalp or hair twiddling	☐	☐	☐
pacing the floor	☐	☐	☐
excessive concern with time – either always late or too early	☐	☐	☐
loss of interest with personal appearance	☐	☐	☐
loss of sense of humour	☐	☐	☐
increased lethargy	☐	☐	☐
accident proneness	☐	☐	☐
difficulty in getting to sleep and/or awakening in the morning	☐	☐	☐
difficulty in getting back to sleep	☐	☐	☐

PHYSICAL SYMPTOMS

	RARELY	SOMETIMES	OFTEN
headaches	☐	☐	☐
dry mouth and/or throat	☐	☐	☐
indigestion	☐	☐	☐
nausea	☐	☐	☐
'butterflies' in the stomach	☐	☐	☐
constipation	☐	☐	☐
diarrhoea	☐	☐	☐
unusual gain or loss in weight	☐	☐	☐
unusual gain or loss of appetite	☐	☐	☐
skin problems – eczema, hives, rashes	☐	☐	☐
ulcers	☐	☐	☐
high blood pressure	☐	☐	☐
palpitations	☐	☐	☐
excessive sweating and/or cold sweats	☐	☐	☐
rapid or irregular breathing	☐	☐	☐
tightness in the chest	☐	☐	☐
increased incidence of allergies	☐	☐	☐
frequent colds and/or influenza	☐	☐	☐
premenstrual tension (PMT)	☐	☐	☐
impotence or frigidity	☐	☐	☐

STRESS AND RELAXATION

Signs of stress at work

	RARELY	SOMETIMES	OFTEN
absenteeism	☐	☐	☐
working long hours	☐	☐	☐
unmet deadlines	☐	☐	☐
reduced productivity	☐	☐	☐
conflicts with colleagues	☐	☐	☐
fault-finding of colleagues	☐	☐	☐
dreading going into work	☐	☐	☐
resentment over pay	☐	☐	☐
inability to take criticism	☐	☐	☐
boredom	☐	☐	☐
frustration	☐	☐	☐
not tackling difficult jobs	☐	☐	☐
giving excuses	☐	☐	☐
feeling unappreciated	☐	☐	☐
resenting, avoiding and/or disliking the boss	☐	☐	☐
lack of communication with colleagues	☐	☐	☐
disliking your job	☐	☐	☐
taking work home	☐	☐	☐
lunchtime drinking	☐	☐	☐
inability to delegate	☐	☐	☐

Signs of stress at home

	RARELY	SOMETIMES	OFTEN
feelings of isolation	☐	☐	☐
lack of privacy	☐	☐	☐
frustration at nothing ever being finished	☐	☐	☐
boredom	☐	☐	☐
feeling unappreciated	☐	☐	☐
resentment at loss of freedom	☐	☐	☐
attempting to be superwoman	☐	☐	☐
lack of patience with the children	☐	☐	☐
nagging and/or subservience to the partner	☐	☐	☐
feelings of hostility	☐	☐	☐
anxiety	☐	☐	☐
resentment over unequal work loads	☐	☐	☐
loss of interest with personal appearance	☐	☐	☐
lethargy	☐	☐	☐
exhaustion	☐	☐	☐
over-concern with petty details	☐	☐	☐
never having time for yourself	☐	☐	☐
bouts of crying	☐	☐	☐
menstrual problems	☐	☐	☐
lack of enjoyable exercise and/or hobbies	☐	☐	☐

STRESS AND RELAXATION

RELAXATION TECHNIQUES

Different techniques are good for different types of personality and general character. Most people discover what helps them relax and reduces the stress of their daily lives fairly quickly, though there is an insidious tendency to convince ourselves that we will do something tomorrow, later or as soon as a particular crisis is over. This is a deceptive philosophy because tomorrow's best intentions have a way of being put off until yet another tomorrow. Meanwhile continuing stress takes its painful toll of your health and the peace of mind of your family and your friends.

Relaxation Tips

Laugh and smile
both release tension, ease difficult situations, relieve embarrassment and diffuse temper. They lighten up your face and dissolve the lines caused by frowns and tension, making you more attractive to others in an instant: it is extremely difficult for someone to feel annoyed when faced with a smile. Laughter renews hope and helps you to view problems in a more positive and objective way.

Walk tall
doing so will almost certainly fool others, and may eventually fool you. Also, it is more difficult to feel depressed and unsure of yourself if you are holding your head high to face the world.

Be realistic
it is no good trying to alter your basic personality; learn to manage it, and to utilize its strengths and accept its weaknesses.

Live in the present
we should learn from our past mistakes but should not carry them around with us. Holding on to past errors is as futile as refusing to let go of an unwieldy suitcase full of outgrown clothes.

Learn to say "no"
both at work and at home, to the children, to your partner and to your boss. You are no good to anyone when you are exhausted, resentful and over-stretched. People will respect you more if you are straightforward and decisive.

Find time to pamper yourself
do not wait for others to suggest that you do so, because you might wait too long, and you know what you like and need. Insist on your own chosen method: it might be a hot bath, a brisk walk in the rain, a good book or an evening chatting to a friend.

Take exercise
any form of exercise is useful for reducing any sudden increase in tension or stress and setting the body back on to an even keel. Go for a walk, take a swim, dance, play tennis or scrub the kitchen floor.

Respect your own sexuality
sex with the right person is a wonderful way of releasing tension and making one feel needed, desired and attractive.

Stop worrying
either about real or imagined problems. Worrying never achieves anything but heartache, lines on your face and sleepless nights. This is easier said than done, true – but try practising certain tricks to prevent your mind from dwelling on any one problem: watch a comedy; play a complicated game of patience; cook a new and difficult dish; or read a challenging book.

Take pleasure in little things
look out for simple, everyday occurences and relish them: a smile on a child's face; a funny hairstyle; a chance meeting; an unexpected compliment, a joke; a beautiful sunset.

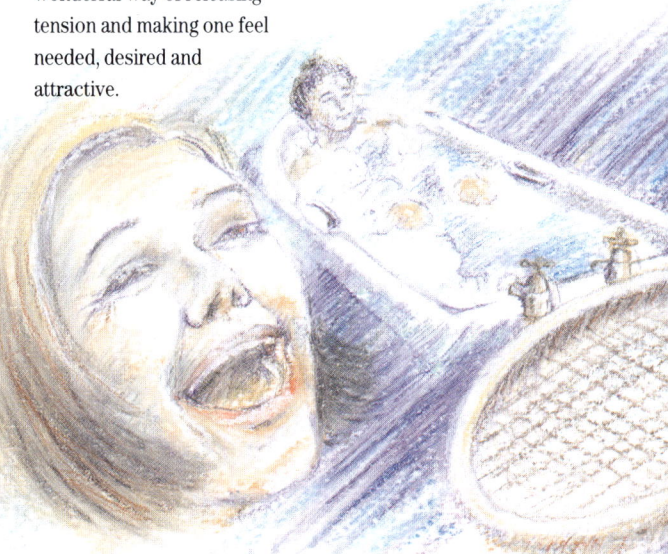

STRESS AND RELAXATION

Learn to know your own priorities

at home, at work and in social situations, try to strike a balance between the imperatives of these three basic aspects of a healthy life. In each area, pay attention to the important things first, because the stress of 'unfinished business' is usually worse than solving the problem. Avoid using trivialities to put off confronting important issues.

Stimulate your mind

if you have a repetitive and boring job, try to change your job to one that suits your personality, because an unsatisfactory and undemanding job can cause a considerable amount of stress. In the mean time take up an exciting hobby, join a club or take a course.

Plan ahead for your retirement

join local organizations, for example, or take up part-time voluntary work. Once retired plan your day, not forgetting time for yourself, until the change from organized work to voluntary discipline has become a habit.

Recognize when to ask for professional help

we all have different stress levels. It is not a sign of weakness to suffer from stress, but more often a sign of overwhelming willpower and determination not to give in or stubbornness in admitting that one is not perfect and invincible.

Personal Programmes

The pages that follow give a number of examples of typically stressful lifestyles from the main decades of adult life: the 20s, 30s, 40s, 50s and 60s. Each decade brings its own particular circumstances, each of which can cause stress; and examples of different problems are given for each one. Of course, not everyone will suffer from these lifestyle scenarios, and, in general, they have been exaggerated here to make a point.

In each case, a personal relaxation programme is prescribed. This will not itself banish the problems – in most cases that are described, only basic and wide-ranging changes in the subject's personal circumstances will give rise to anything that is remotely like a 'cure'. However, following the programmes suggested would enable the subjects to relieve some of symptoms of stress and tension, aid relaxation, and so help the subject (or you) to make rational, considered decisions that can help break the vicious circle of stress.

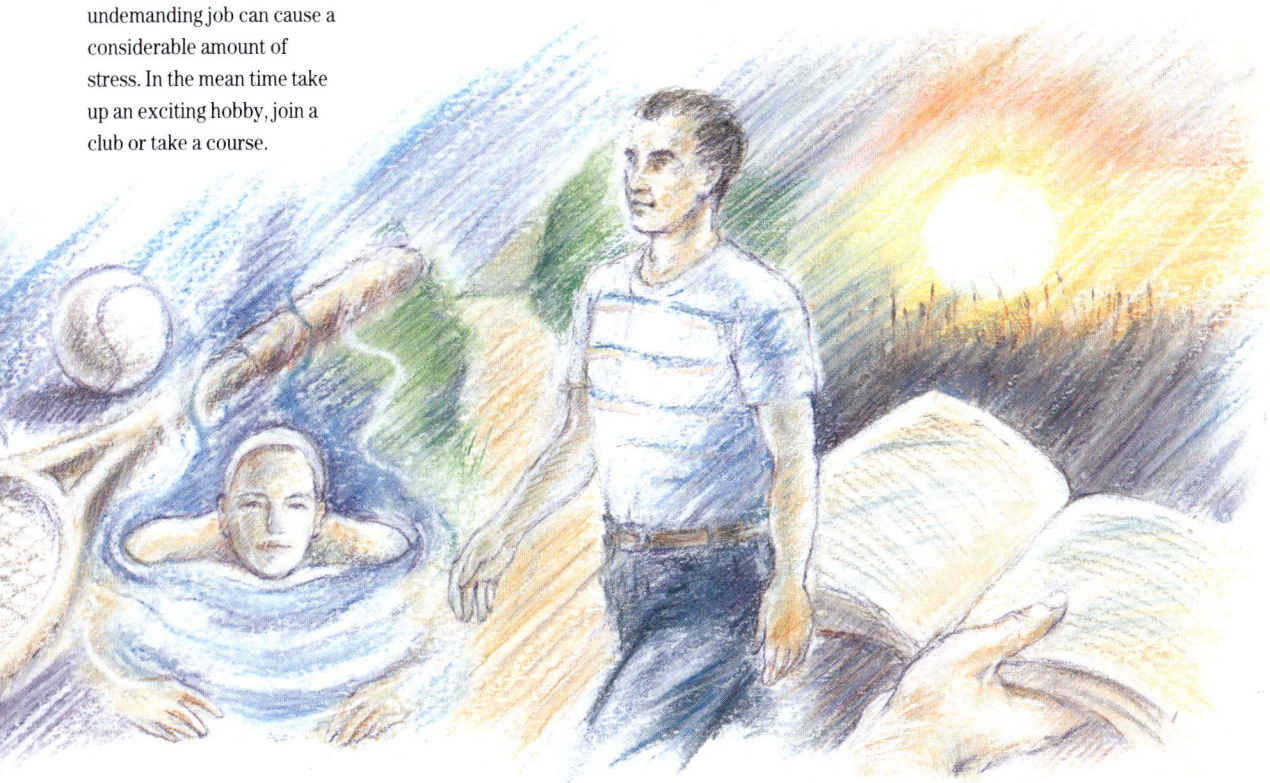

STRESS AND RELAXATION

THE TWENTIES

At the same time as adapting to a new lifestyle, either away from the security of home or of college, people in their twenties are adjusting to their own emergent personalities: they are becoming independent individuals with their own ambitions and requirements but they miss the support they have had. The stress this creates may well increase when he or she starts to experience the clash between personal ideals and dreams and the realities of life.

Typical questions that concern people in their twenties are: Who am I? What am I doing? Where am I going? Will people like me? Am I attractive to the opposite sex? Will someone love me? Such underlying insecurities are often heightened by familial or social expectations.

The way an individual reacts to these pressures depends on his or her personality and background. An extrovert may ignore the problem and concentrate on 'getting on' in life, not allowing time to relax, so that unresolved insecurities and stresses may surface later in life. On the other hand, introverts may worry so much about their real and imaginary problems and fears that they never allow their own positive personalities to develop and flourish.

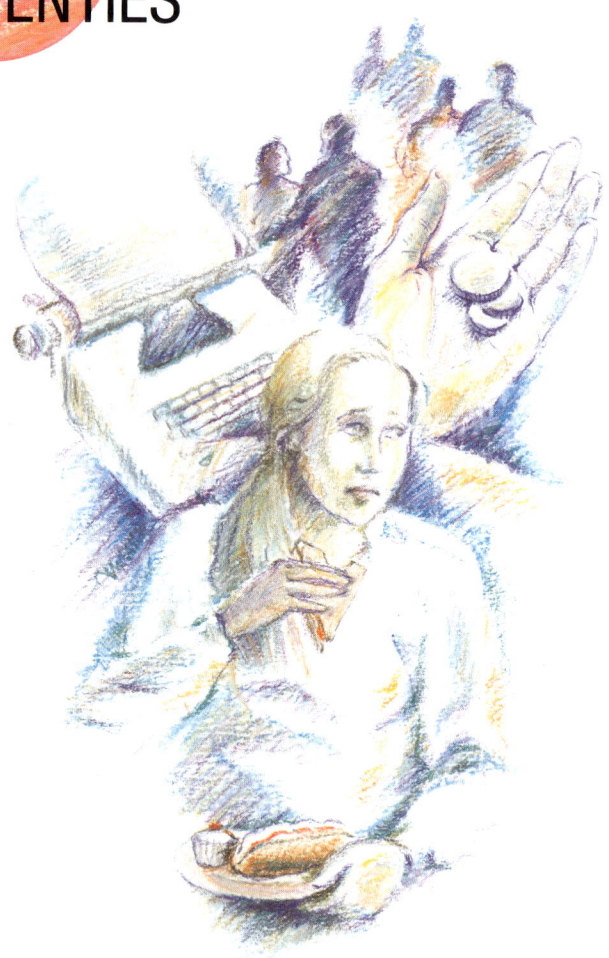

Lifestyles

Andrea – is a 22-year-old secretary. She attended a local secretarial college, then found a job in a large company in a big city, working in the secretarial pool. Andrea's work is repetitive and boring, and there is little contact with anyone outside the other members of the pool. She shares an apartment with three other girls in a quiet, run-down area of town. At first, Andrea was happy with her new life – she revelled in the chatter at work, her new-found freedom from home and her financial independence. This euphoria wore off all too quickly. After paying the rent, she has little money. She feels that her friends only talk about themselves and do not seem interested in her, and as soon as they found boyfriends, she was almost ignored. Without a boyfriend herself and an almost non-existent social life, Andrea feels lonely; she misses her friends, her family and home, where she felt secure and appreciated.

A slim girl when she came to town, Andrea has now started to eat too much and put on weight. Disgusted with her own lack of control, Andrea diets drastically for a few days, and then her body's craving for food and her loneliness triggers an eating binge. A vicious circle of bingeing and starving has developed. Her body reacts to this stress and she is often constipated; her periods are irregular; and she has become moody, with great emotional swings between extrovert behaviour, slight hysteria and gaiety, and bouts of despondency and crying when she hides herself away.

Andrea dislikes her own weakness, her body, her work and her lack of a social life, but does not feel capable of altering it. She is too proud to admit her worries and fears to her family, always claiming that she loves her job, has an active social life and is happy. Her parents do not believe her, but since they cannot breach the new barriers that she has erected round her life the relationship is under strain, so Andrea visits home less and less and feels guilty and homesick.

PERSONAL RELAXATION PROGRAMME
Basic relaxation technique (p56)
Nutritional medicine (p130) and/or naturopathy (p134)
Autosuggestion (p120) and/or visualization (p122)
Yoga (p110) and/or dance therapy (p147)
Hydrotherapy (p90)

Graham – is a good-looking 24-year-old junior lawyer. He is highly ambitious and from an early age has been determined to have the good things in life, not having to scrimp and save as his parents did.

During the day, Graham works hard, and often stays late – especially if his boss is around – and takes a lot of trouble to make himself popular and indispensable. Outside work, he socializes a great deal, trying to network, and so build up a circle of contacts that might be useful in furthering his career.

Graham gives little thought to his lifestyle or to the stresses that it might be producing. He ignores his often aggressive behaviour and the tantrums he displays when he does not get his own way. He is unconcerned about his inability to relax after a day's work, and does not notice that he finds it difficult to accept criticism even though he often finds fault with others.

Graham acknowledges that he is a heavy drinker; he often suffers from heartburn, as well as odd aches and pains, but he is confident he will eventually cut down his alcohol consumption and live a more relaxed life – when he has achieved his goals.

PERSONAL RELAXATION PROGRAMME
Basic relaxation technique (p56)
Hydrotherapy (p90)
Massage (p72) and/or aromatherapy (p80)
Biofeedback (p129) and/or autosuggestion (p120)
Self-hypnosis (p126)
Music therapy (p148)

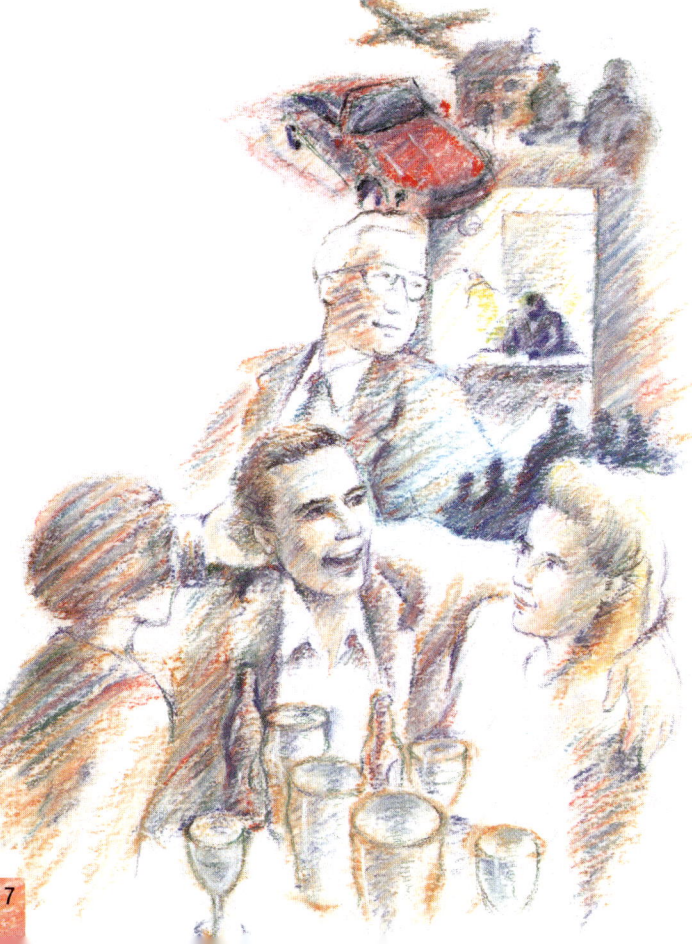

STRESS AND RELAXATION

Jane – is a recently married 26-year-old woman with a young baby. On getting married, she gave up her job in hospital and moved away to an area where she had no friends. Jane wanted to find a new job as a way of meeting new people, but became pregnant before she could do so.

At first, Jane was happy: the excitement of having a home of her own to organize, her new husband and the prospect of the baby all made her feel secure and grown-up. But after the initial euphoria of the baby's birth had worn off, Jane became depressed. Her husband is ambitious and works long hours, leaving their small house early each morning and arriving home late, often exhausted and irritable. He plays sport most Saturdays and goes out for a drink with his friends after the game.

Jane is exhausted by the perpetual demands of the baby, developing constant backache and suffering frequent headaches. She finds the broken nights difficult and has trouble getting back to sleep. She also worries about how the baby is doing, but has few friends and no family nearby with whom she can talk things over. Her husband thinks that all women instinctively know how to care for a baby and Jane feels he is not very understanding or supportive and resents his lack of help.

Jane's new life seems to be one of perpetual tiredness, loss of freedom and the repetitive boredom of household chores. She has started to resent her husband's freedom and unchanged lifestyle but, instead of talking to him about it, she nags, complains or bursts into tears, and is an emotional see-saw. Jane has also lost interest in sex, lost her sense of humour and does not bother much with her personal appearance.

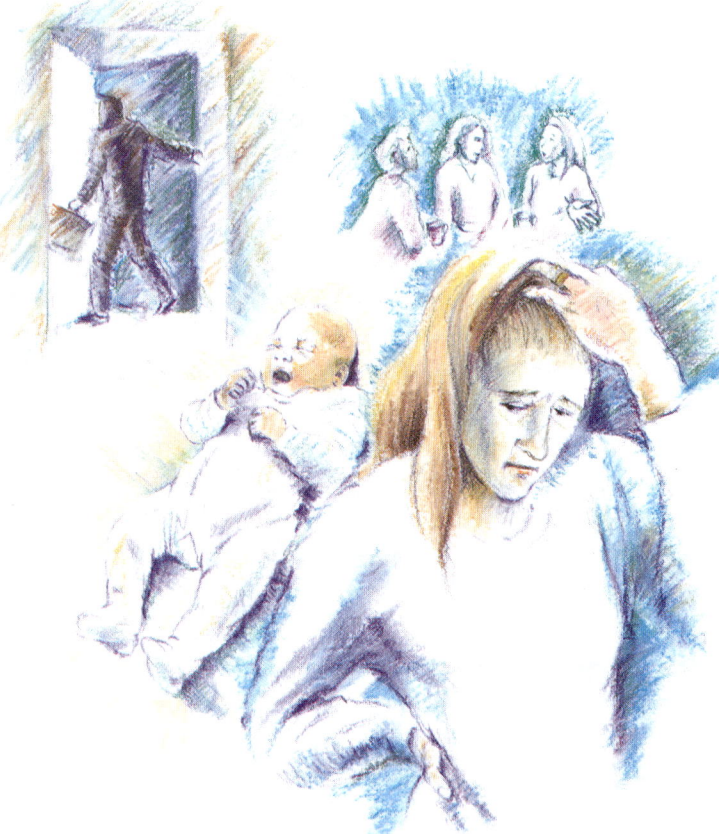

PERSONAL RELAXATION PROGRAMME
Basic relaxation technique (p56)
Improving posture (p64) and/or Alexander technique (p102)
Yoga (p110) and/or meditation (p118)
Music (p148) and/or dance therapy (p147)
Massage (p72) and/or aromatherapy (p80)
Colour (p142) and/or art therapy (p150)

THE TWENTIES

Vivien – is a 28-year-old teacher at an inner-city school. He took up his post straight from training college, which he left as an idealist, determined to be a good teacher and to help all his pupils achieve their own potential whatever the cost to himself.

After a couple of years, Vivien has become disillusioned with unruly pupils, who have little interest in education; lethargic, cynical colleagues; the monolithic, bureaucratic education system; and uncaring or complaining parents. His first solution was to distance himself from his colleagues, but he soon started to criticize both them and the whole educational system. Now he is bitter about their apparent lack of appreciation of his efforts and resentful about his salary, compared to some of his friends outside teaching.

Instead of facing the realities of the situation and coping with them, Vivien has started to arrive late, unprepared for the day's classes; he fails to mark papers and generally does as little extra-curricular work as he can get away with.

Vivien shows many of the signs of being under great emotional stress. He is irritable, lethargic, lazy and hostile; he cannot concentrate well and his memory has deteriorated; he sleeps badly and finds it difficult to get up in the morning – in fact, he finds it difficult to do anything. He often has headaches, there is a tic in his eye, and he is losing weight. His friends have started to avoid him, as he is moody, envious and bad-tempered.

PERSONAL RELAXATION PROGRAMME
Basic relaxation technique (p56)
Visualization (p122) and/or autosuggestion (p120)
Music (p148) and/or art therapy (p150)
Yoga (p110) and/or breathing techniques (p60)
Homoeopathy (p138) and/or Bach flower technique (p141)

STRESS AND RELAXATION

THE THIRTIES

Many people feel fairly relaxed and in control of their destiny in their thirties: they are young, fit and unconcerned about old age, and they are over the insecurities of the twenties. Many have to come to terms with the realities of their own personalities, their intellects and the world around them. But others often feel that they made the wrong decision about their career or their marriage. When other considerations – such as family responsibilities or lack of financial security – prevent them from making any changes, they feel bitter and frustrated.

A woman who married young and stayed at home often feels that she has never developed her own personality and potential and has ambivalent feelings towards her dependency on her husband and her children's dependency on her. Men and women who have careers often become disillusioned and resentful if their rewards do not match expectations, or develop the signs of tension and stress from the pressure that they put themselves under.

Lifestyles

Lynette – is a highly successful career woman in her late thirties. She is financially independent and always looks smart. Her married woman friends envy Lynette her freedom and independence, and her male friends find her slightly intimidating, though attractive.

Lynette is inclined to be a loner and has never needed a permanent relationship or a family. Suddenly, though, she has realized that with each passing year her opportunity to become a mother (and, as she is so often reminded, to give her mother a grandchild) is lessened; she might have to spend the rest of her life on her own. She also feels tired of being a woman in a man's world, with the need to be at once assertive and dominant but always attractive and feminine; she secretly thinks that it might be quite nice to have someone to look after her.

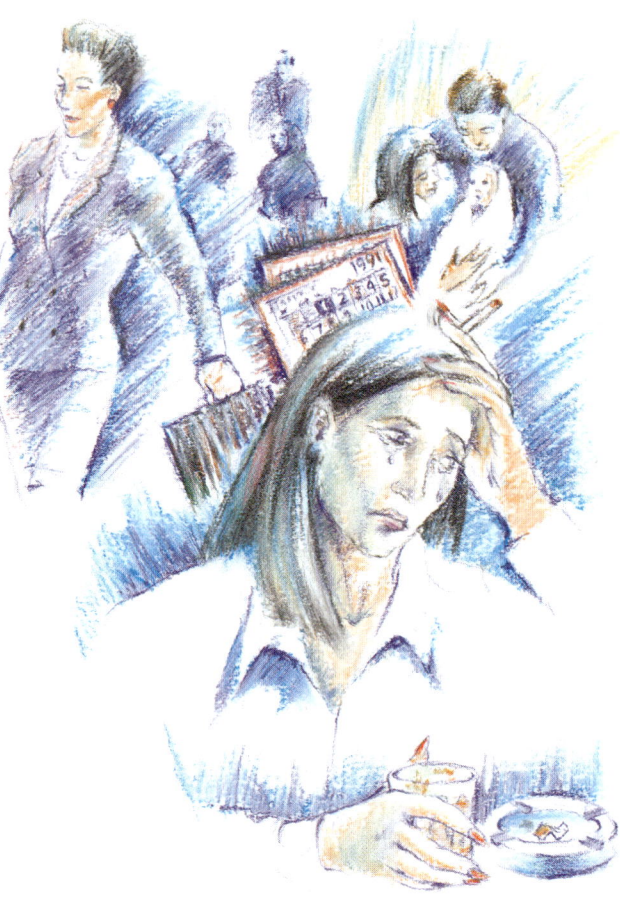

Lynette has become increasingly anxious that she is unable to control her emotions. She sleeps badly, often waking in a hot sweat after bad dreams. She tends to cry for no apparent reason when alone, so she socializes aggressively and has more casual sexual relationships – though she enjoys them less. Her smoking and drinking have increased as her productivity and concentration at work have diminished – she has started to find it harder to make decisions and dreads having to go into work.

> **PERSONAL RELAXATION PROGRAMME**
> Basic relaxation technique (p56)
> Yoga (p110) and/or meditation (p118)
> Massage (p72) and/or aromatherapy (p80)
> Music (p148) and/or dance therapy (p147)
> Visualization (p122) and/or autogenic therapy (p121)
> Self-hypnosis (p126) and/or breathing (p60)

Kirsten – is in her early thirties, a wife with two children, who had to return to work as a part-time receptionist in a doctor's office for financial reasons. She is a trained nurse, but stopped work for her first child.

Kirsten is well-organized and enjoyed her work and the feelings of independence that it gave her – at first. She takes the children to school in the morning before work, shopping in her lunch break. After work, she collects the children and goes home to do all the household chores. The weekends are an endless round, in which she finishes all the jobs left over from the previous week. She has slowly realized that she is very dissatisfied with her life.

Kirsten is frustrated at not being able to do the job for which she was trained. At work, she worries about her children and the house; at home she feels resentful because her children and husband prevent her from resuming her nursing career – then she feels guilty about her resentment. She also feels guilty and worries whenever one of the children falls ill – either because she takes time off work and so earns less money, or because the child is with someone else. Kirsten's husband still feels that he is the main bread winner, and she believes that he is unappreciative of her efforts.

Kirsten has begun to find it increasingly difficult to

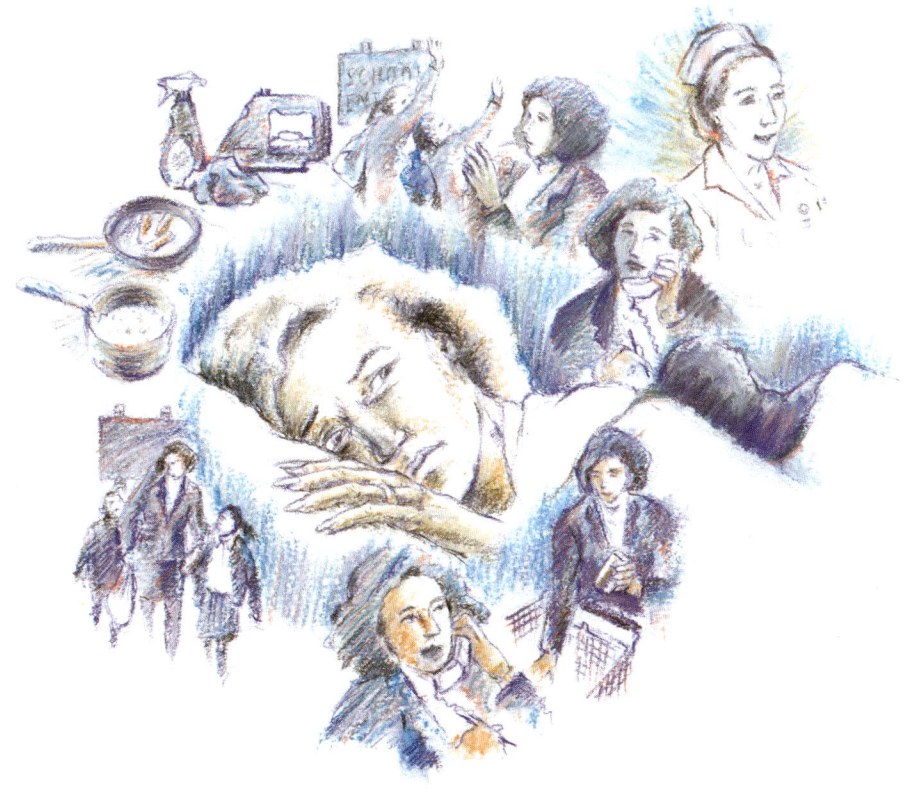

STRESS AND RELAXATION

relax. She is always tense and irritable, and has sudden feelings of panic, with tightness in her chest. She cannot get to sleep – the lists of chores for the next day whirl around her head. She has started to shout at her children one minute and ignore them the next. Her relationship with her husband has deteriorated as her feelings of hostility at his lack of understanding increase. Kirsten stays in her subservient role, though, never requesting help, and rarely discussing her problems or feelings with him. He is confused by her changes of mood.

PERSONAL RELAXATION PROGRAMME
Basic relaxation technique (p56)
Breathing techniques (p60)
Hydrotherapy (p90) and/or aromatherapy (p80)
Colour (p142) and/or smell therapy (p82)
Yoga (p110) and/or dance therapy (p147)
Visualization (p122) and/or autosuggestion (p120)

David – is an entrepreneur in his mid thirties, who runs his own small company. Married with children, David has always lived hard and worked long hours – he is ambitious and determined and wants to provide the best for his wife and children. His only relaxation is to go out for a drink after work, before returning home and slumping in front of the television.

Since an economic downturn has affected his business, David has started to sleep badly. He often wakes at night in a cold sweat and with a pounding heart, and gets up in the morning feeling unrefreshed and exhausted. At work he is irritable and critical of his staff, and he finds it increasingly difficult to concentrate, or to tackle difficult tasks.

David suffers from severe headaches, as a result of tension in his neck and shoulders, and often grinds his teeth. In response he has started to drink heavily – it is the only way that he can put his problems out of his mind. At home, he is moody and critical, feeling that his family does not appreciate the stress he is under. His relationship with his wife is deteriorating and he has started to look for casual sexual relationships to momentarily relieve his stress.

As David's stress level has increased, he has developed palpitations, indigestion, nausea and heartburn and, for the first time, has become seriously concerned about his health.

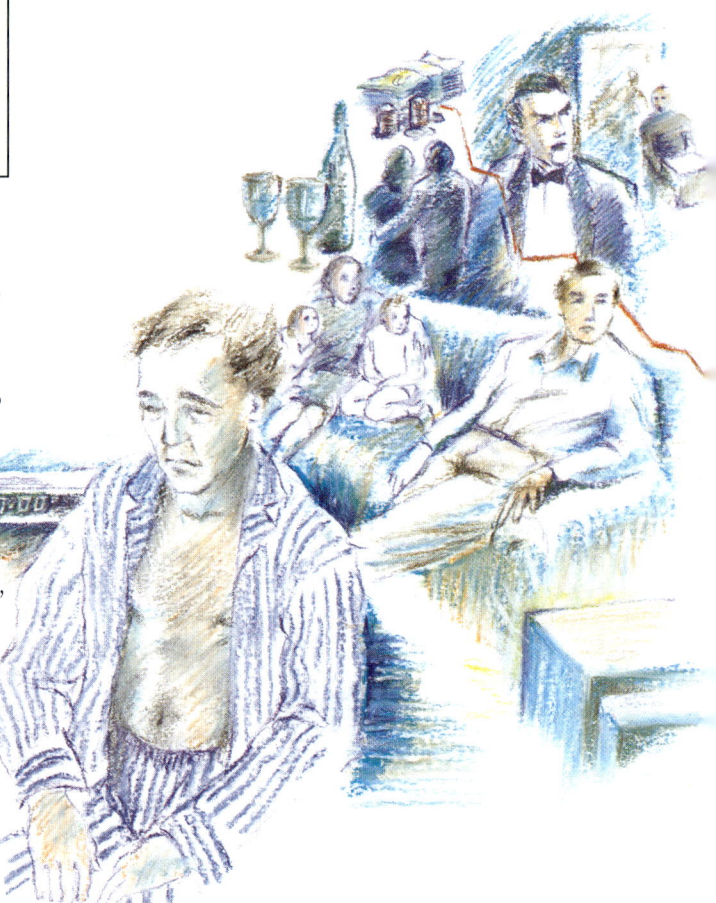

THE THIRTIES

> **PERSONAL RELAXATION PROGRAMME**
> Basic relaxation programme (p56)
> Naturopathy (p134) and/or nutritional medicine (p130)
> Biofeedback (p129) and/or visualization (p122)
> Self-hypnosis (p126) and/or autosuggestion (p120)
> Massage (p72) and/or hydrotherapy (p90)
> Music therapy (p148)
> TENS therapy (p96)

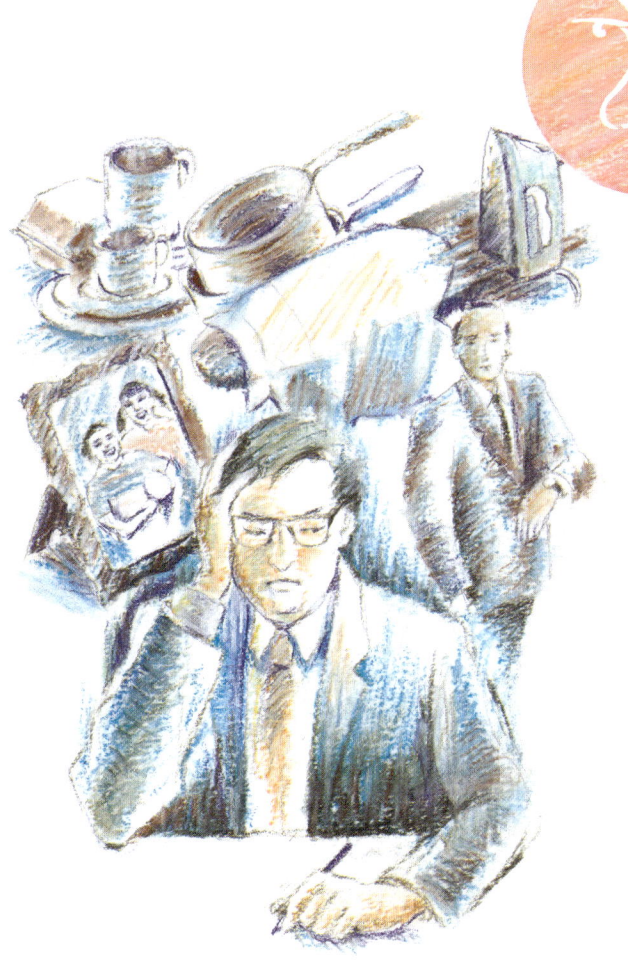

Andrew – is recently divorced, in his late thirties, and now lives on his own in a small flat. Andrew pays alimony and child maintenance, and though earning a reasonable wage, he feels extremely bitter at having to pay out what he considers to be too high a percentage of it to support his former family and home.

Andrew dislikes having to live on his own and having to cope with his own domestic arrangements. He desperately misses his children and finds his weekend outings with them unsatisfactory and frequently over-emotional; he feels both guilty and a failure as a father.

Andrew is often morose and emotional at the office and lacks any interest in or enthusiasm for his work. He is often late for deadlines and makes silly mistakes. Andrew is aware that his boss, at first sympathetic, is becoming increasingly annoyed with his lack of achievement; as a result, he worries about his future and the safety of his job within the company.

Andrew blames his former wife for the divorce and feels that he can never trust or like another woman again. He has lost all interest in social life and sexual relationships. He has put on a lot of weight since the divorce, so feels fat and unattractive, but cannot summon up enough energy to do anything about it. He sleeps fitfully, suffers from colds, and has episodes in which his whole body seems to ache. In short, Andrew feels he is a failure as a man, a husband and a father.

> **PERSONAL RELAXATION PROGRAMME**
> Basic relaxation technique (p56)
> Alexander technique (p102)
> Feldenkrais techniques (p108)
> Reflexology (p86) and/or acupressure (p84)
> Self-hypnosis (p126) and/or visualization therapy (p122)
> Autogenic (p121) and/or autosuggestion (p120)
> Homoeopathy (p138) and/or Bach flower techniques (p141)
> Music (p148) and/or art therapy (p150)
> Naturopathy (p134) and/or herbalism (p136)

STRESS AND RELAXATION

The Forties

The forties can be the most stressful decade of life since people often have children at home, the divorce rate has increased; and economic and career pressures are more severe than ever.

Lifestyles

Sylvie – is a 42-year-old divorced woman with four children. After the divorce, she moved which meant that her children had to change schools and no longer lived close to their friends. Sylvie went to work full-time. For 15 years, she had worked part-time as a designer – mainly to support her husband in his budding career – and cared for the children; this was very much the role that she had expected to fulfil. She felt nervous about being able to cope with the children, the house and a new job on her own.

Sylvie's previous company, an advertising agency, gave her a job which she enjoys, but she soon discovered that she needed a nanny. At work, Sylvie has to meet strict deadlines and is expected to put in the same overtime and appear as well-dressed as her colleagues. The children resent her going to work full-time, miss their father and their friends and are frequently difficult at home and at school. The children's schools expect Sylvie to go to meetings and functions and to help the children with their homework. Individual nannies have rarely stayed for long, often giving little notice, and the changes are unsettling.

Although Sylvie receives a maintenance payment from her ex-husband, she has to give half of her monthly wage to the nanny. As she is no longer fully in charge of the house, the bills have increased and she spends more money on convenience food and treats for the children. She feels inadequate as a mother and provider.

As a result, Sylvie is perpetually exhausted. She has little time to rebuild her own life and she is still bitter about the divorce and resentful about her former husband's seemingly easy lifestyle and new-found freedom in his attractive new flat.

Sylvie is heading for a complete emotional and physical breakdown. She suffers from feelings of hopelessness and helplessness; complete panic alternates with anger, envy and resentment. She has increased symptoms of premenstrual tension and bouts of uncontrollable self-pity and despair. She has frequent headaches and backache, and suffers from indigestion and flatulence. She is aging fast.

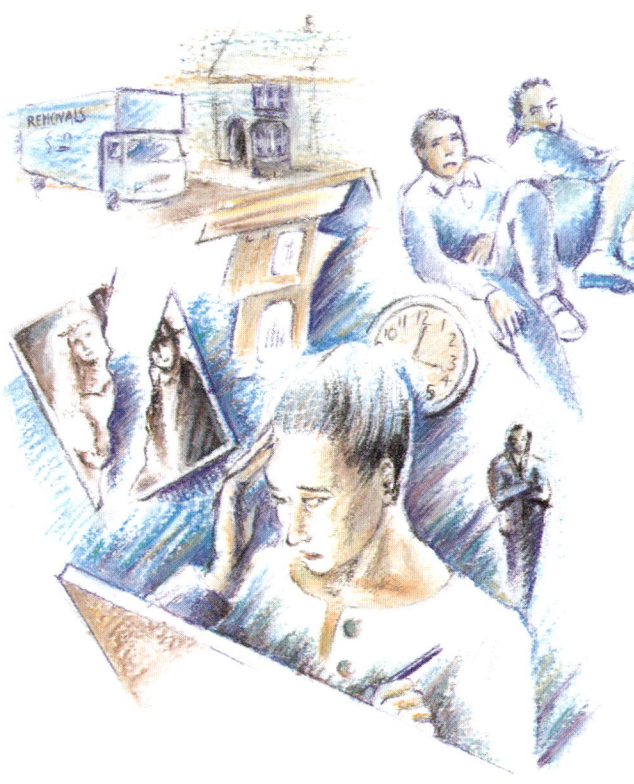

THE FORTIES

> **PERSONAL RELAXATION PROGRAMME**
> Basic relaxation technique (p56)
> Breathing techniques (p60)
> Massage (p72) and/or aromatherapy (p80)
> Acupressure (p84) and/or reflexology (p86)
> Homoeopathy (p138)
> Self-hypnosis (p126) and/or visualization (p122)
> Autosuggestion (p120)
> Hydrotherapy (p90)
> Music (p148) and/or dance therapy (p147)

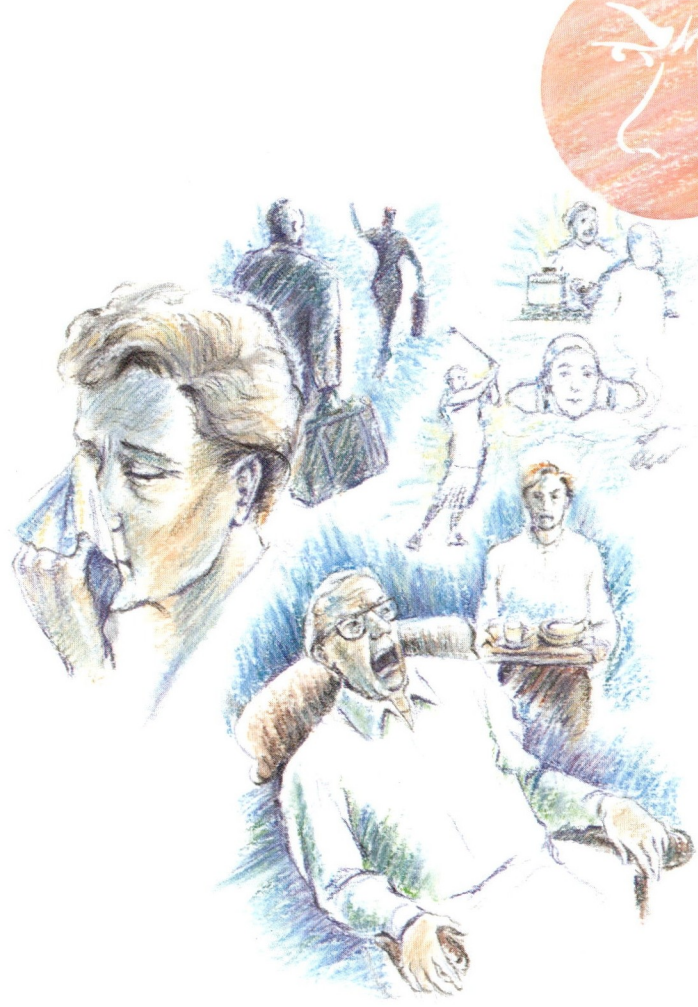

Sue – is 47, and was starting to enjoy a certain freedom in her life. The family was financially secure, the children had left home, and she was free to join various clubs and work as a part-time volunteer for charity. She was still fit and played golf once or twice a week.

Suddenly, Sue's mother died and after the funeral her father came to stay. At first, it was purely a visit – an opportunity to get over his bereavement before returning home. But it soon became clear that Sue's father was not capable of looking after himself. Her family put pressure on Sue and her husband to care for her father, and since they had no vital commitments she felt obliged to agree. Her husband, who was often away on business, felt that it was not really his concern or decision.

Sue began to feel resentful at being tied down once more. She had to give up her charity work and lost contact with many of her friends as her father's health deteriorated. He became more demanding and unsatisfied – nothing she did appeared to be right. More annoyingly, he always behaved well in front of visitors and her husband, who could not understand why she complained so incessantly. Sue felt isolated and unappreciated; she became frustrated, withdrawn and disinterested in the house and herself.

At about the same time, Sue's husband started to come home even later than usual and seemed to have more meetings and weekends away, he appeared to have lost all interest in her. Sue is convinced that her husband is having an affair. She has become hysterical, suspicious, irrational and demanding. The more her husband tries to reassure her, the more convinced she is that she is correct. She cries frequently and suffers from insomnia and bouts of diarrhoea. She blames her father, distrusts her husband and dislikes herself.

> **PERSONAL RELAXATION PROGRAMME**
> Basic relaxation technique (p56)
> Aromatherapy (p80) and/or hydrotherapy (p90)
> Alexander technique (p102) and/or yoga (p110)
> Music (p148) and/or dance therapy (p147)
> Colour (p142) and/or art therapy (p150)

STRESS AND RELAXATION

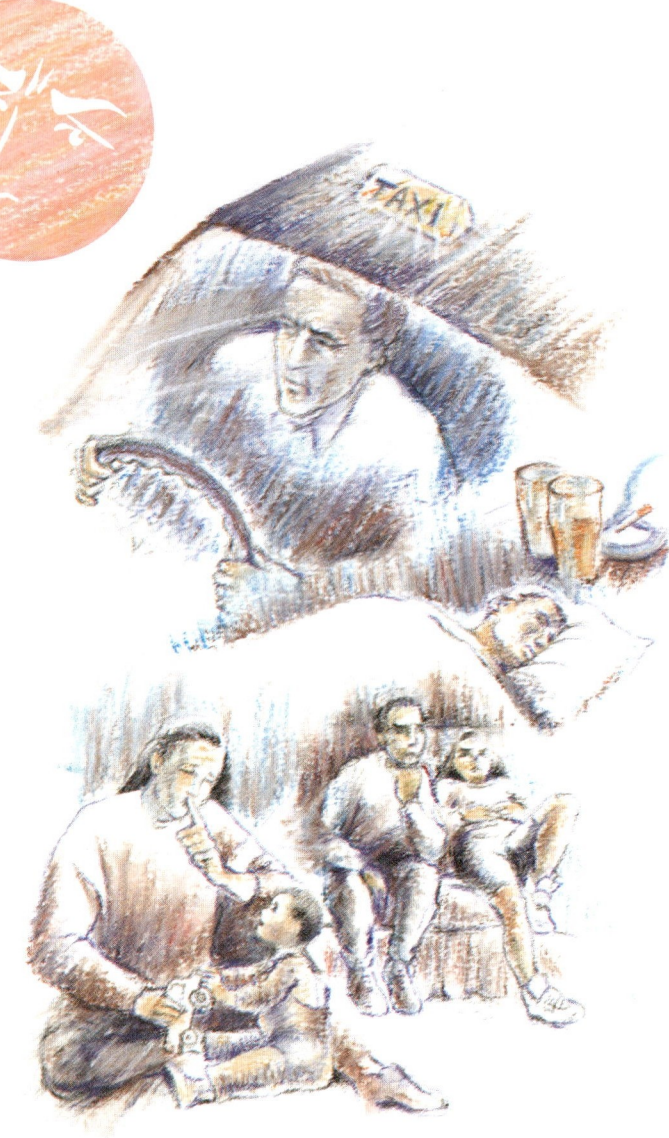

day, Peter saw little of his children or his wife, who became resentful of having to keep the young children quiet during the day and disgruntled with their lack of any social life.

Peter's step-children blame him for the break-up of their parents' marriage and are surly and insolent. When he tries to remonstrate with them, their mother always supports her children against him, leading to frequent arguments and tension.

Peter has become disillusioned with his new family and resentful at its lack of attention to his needs. He finds it impossible to relax when he is driving – he tends to sit with hunched shoulders, gripping the steering wheel fiercely, and loses his temper with other drivers, as well as becoming increasingly rude to his passengers. These problems have led to severe back and neck pain, and sometimes his breathing is difficult and irregular; he sweats continually and complains of wind and constipation. To cope he has started smoking once more, and is drinking in secret.

Peter – is in his late forties, on his second marriage, with two step-children and a young child by his second wife. He was made redundant after the collapse of his first marriage and began to drink heavily and consistently. He was told by his physician to stop drinking completely and find an unstressful job.

Peter found it difficult to find a new job and ended up working as a taxi driver. He found this boring and unrewarding, but it was essential that he persevered – often working unsociable long hours at night – in order to support his new family. As he often slept during the

> **PERSONAL RELAXATION PROGRAMME**
> Basic relaxation technique (p56)
> Improving posture (p64) and/or breathing techniques (p60)
> Alexander technique (p102)
> Naturopathy (p134)
> Visualization (p122) and/or autogenic therapy (p121)
> Biofeedback (p129)
> Music (p148) and/or art therapy (p150)

Francis – is a 43-year-old literary editor on a newspaper. He is in reasonable shape for his age, and still runs occasionally to try and keep fit, but drinks and smokes to excess. He was a lady's man in his youth, but is becoming increasingly concerned that he might be losing both his charm and his ability to attract the opposite sex. He worries about his receeding hairline, grey hair, sagging jaw, and growing paunch. To compensate for this increasing lack of confidence in his appearance, Francis is becoming more extrovert, loud and insensitive to the feelings of others.

At work Francis is increasingly infuriated by his lack of advancement. He knows that he is good and feels bitter when younger people move higher up the ladder. He dislikes his boss and resents the fact that she is a woman. As Francis feels increasingly rejected and neglected, he has begun to lose pride in his work, delivering shoddy, inaccurate copy and missing deadlines. He takes long lunches and often arrives late in the morning.

Francis's dissatisfaction with his work and his dread of middle-age have made him an angry and aggressive man. He is always criticizing others, but brooks no criticism of himself. He has lost both his sense of humour and his sense of proportion, often being irrational and overreacting to the smallest thing. He has started to complain of palpitations and an awareness of his heartbeat. The palms of his hands and his upper lip sweat, he needs to urinate frequently and suffers from indigestion.

> **PERSONAL RELAXATION PROGRAMME**
> Basic relaxation technique (p56)
> Breathing techniques (p60)
> Yoga (p110) and/or meditation (p118)
> Visualization (p122) and/or autosuggestion (p120)
> Music (p148) and/or smell therapy (p82)
> Nutritional medicine (p130) and/or naturopathy (p134)
> Biofeedback (p129)

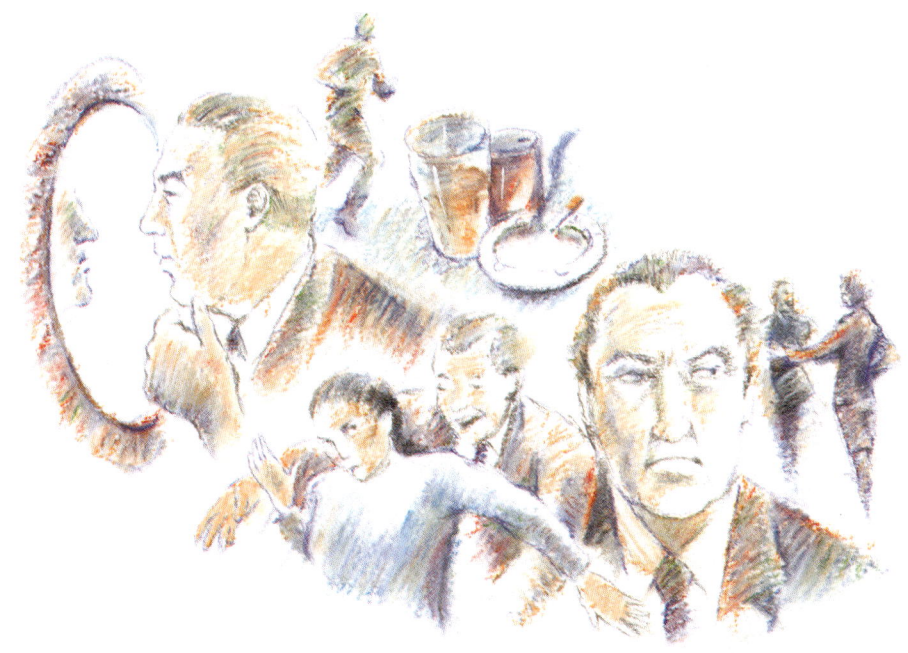

STRESS AND RELAXATION

THE FIFTIES

The fifties can be a time of considerable stress – as much as anything from the realization that you may never achieve your ambition, or the feeling that you may have wasted your opportunities or not fully developed your own personality. Added to this is worry about your children as they leave home to cope on their own, and concern over their disappointments and their failures. There may be guilt, too, about what you perceive as your failings as a parent, or, indeed, a sense of regret if you had no children. Retirement starts to prey on people's minds during the fifties, together with worries about how to cope with old age and the death of friends and relatives. Health can become a problem.

Lifestyles

Eddette – is a housewife in her mid fifties. She has supported her husband in his career by sublimating her desire to his, by maintaining a perfect household and by being an accomplished hostess. The children have all left home and she feels lonely, missing not only their company but her role as a mother. Two of the children live a long way from home and rarely come to visit; the third child is at university, completely wrapped up in his new life and his own needs.

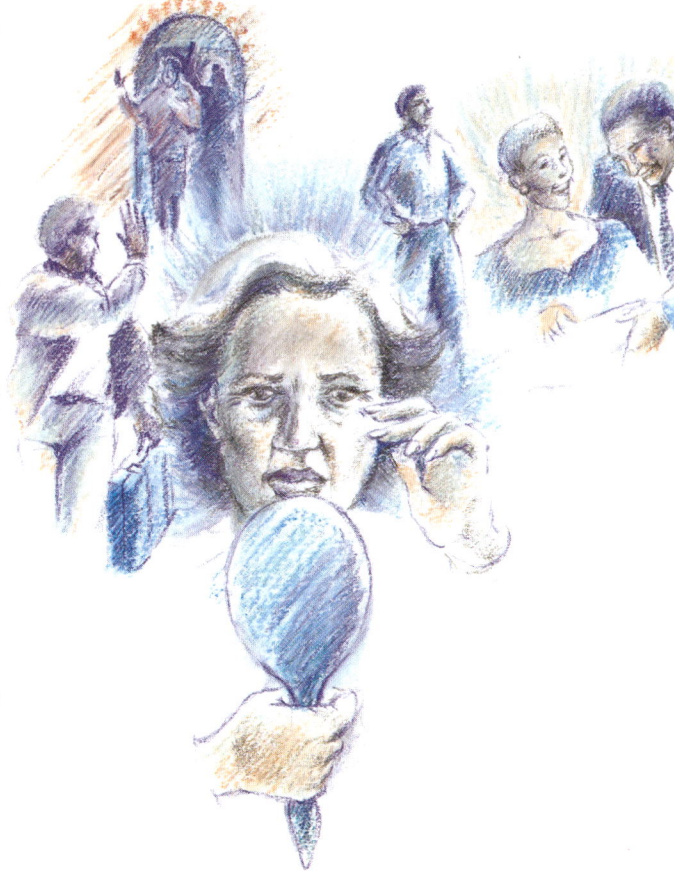

Eddette is also going through the menopause, and suffering from hot flushes, irregular and heavy periods, and occasional urinary tract and vaginal infections. She has uncontrollable mood swings and feels that she is losing control both over her body and her mind. She worries continually about encroaching old age and searches for wrinkles and age spots, sagging skin and new grey hairs – and, of course, she finds them. Her anxiety over her looks is compounded by the fact that her husband, who is a few years younger, is still fit, healthy and energetic.

Eddette has started to wonder what she has achieved in her life – for herself, that is. What has she to show for the last thirty-odd years? Have any of her efforts or sacrifices been appreciated, or even noticed? Will her husband still find her attractive now she is aging, especially when each day he sees young, fresh women who are impressed by his looks, position and power? Eddette feels insecure and vulnerable; her self-esteem is at a low ebb and she has lost the self-confidence and poise that has always been her trade-mark. She feels lethargic and dispirited – as if everything is too much effort. Added to this is the fact that she is increasingly suspicious and irrational, watching for any signs that her husband is losing interest in her. Eddette has become her own worst enemy.

THE FIFTIES

> **PERSONAL RELAXATION PROGRAMME**
> Basic relaxation technique (p56)
> Massage (p72) and aromatherapy (p80)
> Smell therapy (p82)
> Music (p148) and dance therapy (p147)
> Autosuggestion (p120) and/or visualization (p122)
> Yoga (p110) and/or meditation (p118)
> Hydrotherapy (p90)
> Art (p150) and/or colour therapy (p142)

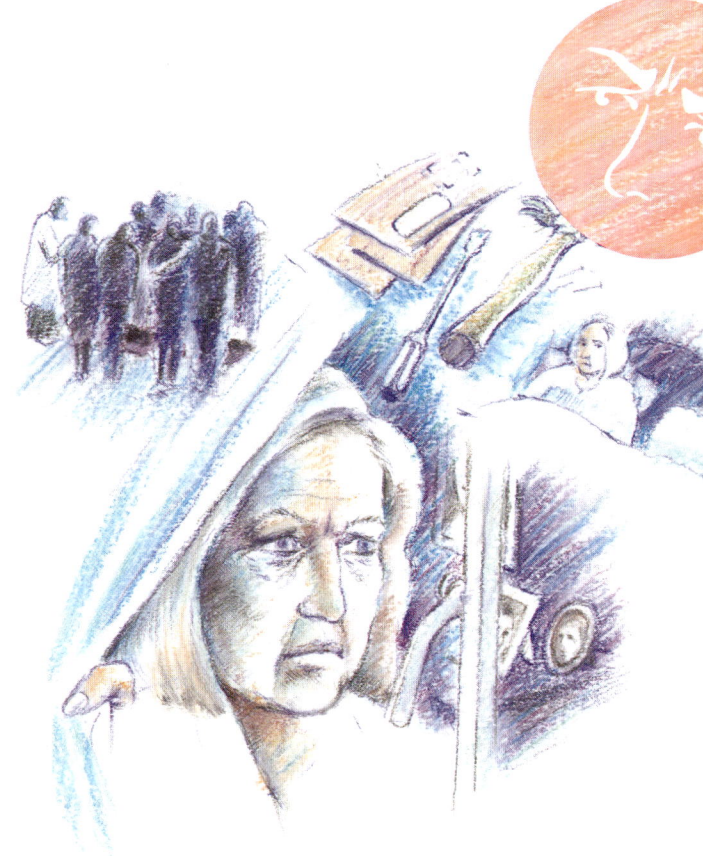

Verity – in her late fifties, has recently lost her husband. Her marriage was a happy one and she feels lost and incomplete without him. She sometimes finds herself feeling angry that he has left her, unprotected, to cope with her grief and her life. She has gradually withdrawn into herself, away from outside social contact, and finds it difficult to get to sleep at night.

Verity also feels bewildered and worried about the practicalities of living, because her husband had always taken care of all their finances – the bills, the mortgage, the insurance – as well as the car and household repairs. She has no idea whether she can manage on a decreased income and worries about her financial security.

An additional source of guilt and worry is that Verity finds it difficult to come to terms with the fact that she still has sexual feelings – these make her feel disloyal to her dead husband and angry with herself. She is also aware that the chances of her finding a new partner at her age are small.

All this worry and stress means that Verity finds it difficult to concentrate. Her memory has become poor and she leaves simple tasks half-complete or untouched; she does not bother to cook proper meals and exists on a poor, uninteresting diet. She is in a vicious circle of decline and needs to re-organize her life on more positive and relaxed lines.

> **PERSONAL RELAXATION PROGRAMME**
> Basic relaxation technique (p56)
> Improving posture (p64) and/or Alexander technique (p102)
> Aromatherapy (p80) and/or smell therapy (p82)
> Homoeopathy (p138) and/or herbalism (p136)
> Naturopathy (p134) and/or nutritional medicine (p130)
> Music (p148) and dance therapy (p147)
> Art therapy (p150)
> Hydrotherapy (p90)

STRESS AND RELAXATION

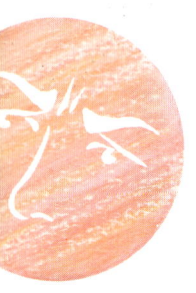

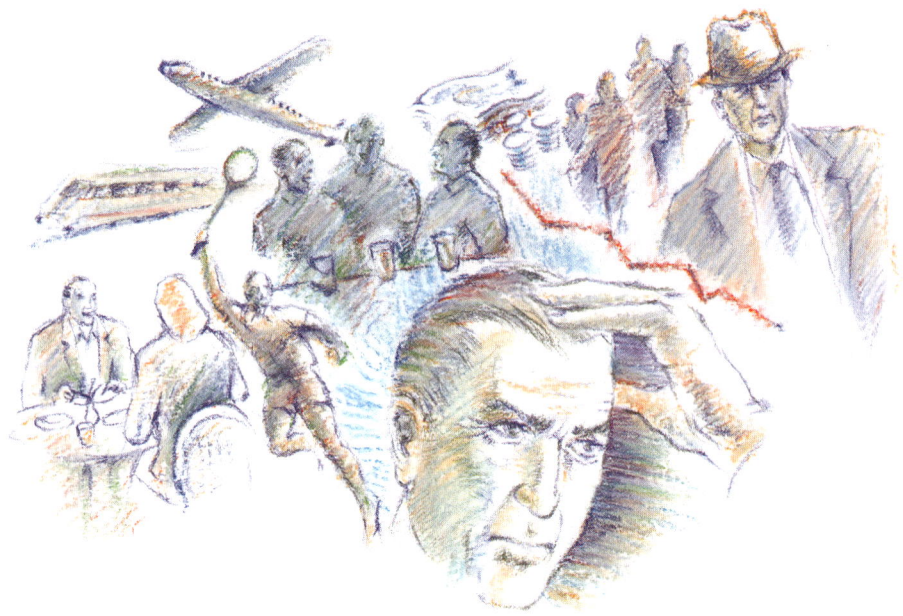

Chris – a divorced man, is now a confirmed bachelor in his mid-fifties who enjoys short-term liaisons with women. He has always worked for himself. Chris has never saved or worried about the future and lives from day to day, surviving on his charm, good looks and social graces.

A good sportsman in his day, Chris is still fit and energetic, favouring the company of younger people – perhaps because they make him forget the inexorable approach of old age. He lives hard, drinking a lot, sleeping little and travelling extensively; in fact, he is running away from the realities of his situation.

With inflation and an economic downturn, Chris is finding it increasingly difficult to maintain his lifestyle and make ends meet. With increasing age, he is not attracting as many women as he used to, and because his friends and acquaintances are all starting to settle down he has to keep finding new friends to impress and charm.

As a result, Chris sleeps badly and wakes early; he loses his temper easily and quickly becomes irritated by any lack of attention from others. He holds grudges and feels bitter about what he wrongly perceives to be betrayal and disloyalty on the part of others. He gets headaches, partly as a result of a recent tendency to grind his teeth and clench his jaw, and has lost his coordination at sport as well as suffering from cramp and odd aches and pains – so he has stopped playing games. In short, Chris resents the onset of old age, is losing his self-confidence and is beginning to fear for a future that looks increasingly bleak.

PERSONAL RELAXATION PROGRAMME
Basic relaxation technique (p56)
Meditation (p118) and/or yoga (p110)
T'ai chi (p98)
Naturopathy (p134) and/or nutritional medicine (p130)
Music (p148) and/or art therapy (p150)

THE FIFTIES

Richard – is in his late fifties, a high-powered business man and owner of a successful company. Richard has always been ambitious, hard, aggressive and ruthless. He pushes himself and his employees hard – they admire but dislike him, and fear his bad temper and emotional outbursts. In town, where he lives during the week, he is often seen with glamorous women, at nightclubs and in restaurants.

Richard's wife is a quiet, subservient woman who stays in the background. Frightened of his irrational moods, she feels little love or respect for him, but stays with him for the position and wealth that he gives her. Their children are spoilt and expect everything in life to be served up on a silver platter – even so, they resent their father's treatment of their mother and feel no admiration for his success, behaviour or wealth.

Richard has never learnt to relax and now the stress he has lived under for so long has started to take its toll. Occasionally he feels sudden breathlessness, with a tightness in his chest, and has suffered from palpitations. His blood pressure is raised and he wakes in the middle of the night in a hot sweat, with disjointed thoughts tumbling through his mind. He finds it increasingly difficult to concentrate at work and worries that he is losing his touch and his control over the company. This, of course, has increased his bad temper and his intolerance of others. As an outlet for his growing stress Richard has started to smoke and drink heavily. At home, he has become more and more sensitive to the fact that he is only tolerated for his money. He feels resentment and anger at having worked so hard for what now appears to be so little reward; he senses that he is on a downward spiral, but cannot break out so he is moody, sarcastic and withdrawn, which exacerbates an already hopeless situation.

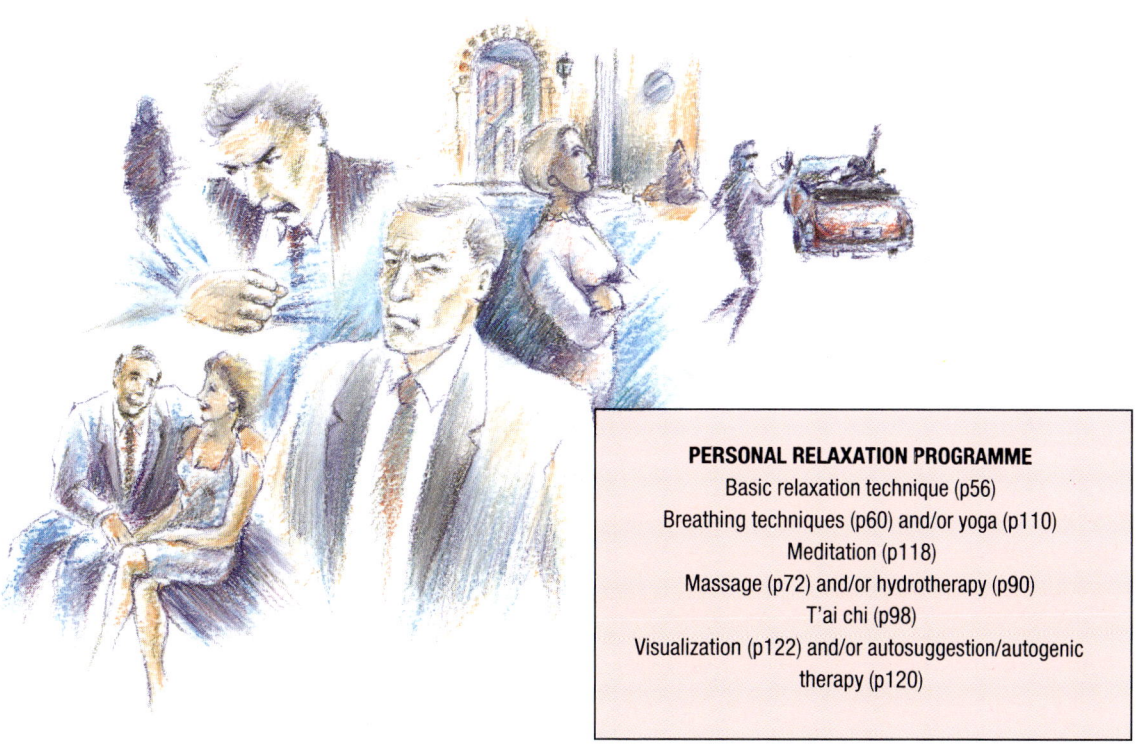

PERSONAL RELAXATION PROGRAMME
Basic relaxation technique (p56)
Breathing techniques (p60) and/or yoga (p110)
Meditation (p118)
Massage (p72) and/or hydrotherapy (p90)
T'ai chi (p98)
Visualization (p122) and/or autosuggestion/autogenic therapy (p120)

STRESS AND RELAXATION

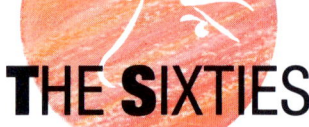

THE SIXTIES

For most people, the seventh decade of life marks a major change in lifestlye. Retirement, paradoxically, is often a time of mounting stress because it becomes increasingly difficult to meet life's challenges as one gets older. Retirement can mean a loss of frendships and social contacts, a loss of a feeling of worth and importance in the scheme of things, and a tendency to feel inadequate and a parasite on society. Boredom and frustration are commonplace; there may also be problems when one now spends all day with one's partner, perhaps for the first time in years.

Before retirement, people often start to dread old age and worry about whether their bodies and financial resources will sustain them. Many have to cope with bereavement and the loss of frequent contact with their children. Failing health, too – either physical or mental, in oneself or in one's spouse – brings its own stresses and strains. On top of all this, the sixties are often the time when we have to come to terms with and accept the damage we have done to our bodies during our lives.

Lifestyles

Sara – is a widow in her mid sixties who lives on her pension. She has been coping well with living on her own, but is becoming increasingly lonely. Many of her friends have moved into old people's homes or moved closer to their children; others have died. One of her children has emigrated – she has never seen her grandchildren; the other lives a hectic life and rarely comes to visit. Sara has always enjoyed good health and taken care of herself, both physically and mentally, but with increasing age she finds she can no longer do just as she likes: her eyesight is failing, and she get headaches if she watches television or reads too much. As a result, she has begun to feel isolated from the outside world and despondent about her lack of social contact.

Sara finds it difficult to combat the tedium of her existence and has started to spend long periods in bed or sitting doing nothing in her chair. Caring for the house, the garden and even herself seems unimportant and irrelevant, especially since she never has any visitors who might appreciate her efforts. Sara is becoming more and more depressed and is taking sleeping pills – both to help her sleep and to pass the time. Constant use has meant that her short-term memory is becoming affected, and she is often confused and forgetful.

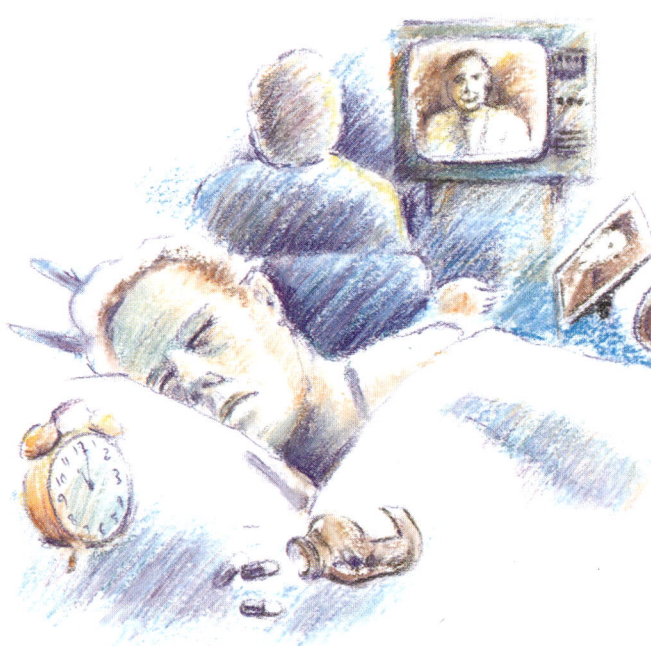

PERSONAL RELAXATION PROGRAMME
Basic relaxation technique (p56)
Aromatherapy (p80) and/or smell therapy (p82)
Art (p150) and colour therapy (p142)
Music (p148) and dance therapy (p147)
Autogenic therapy (p121) and/or visualization (p122)
Yoga (p110)

THE SIXTIES

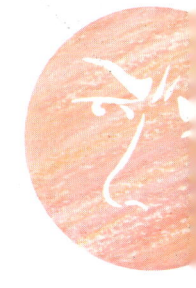
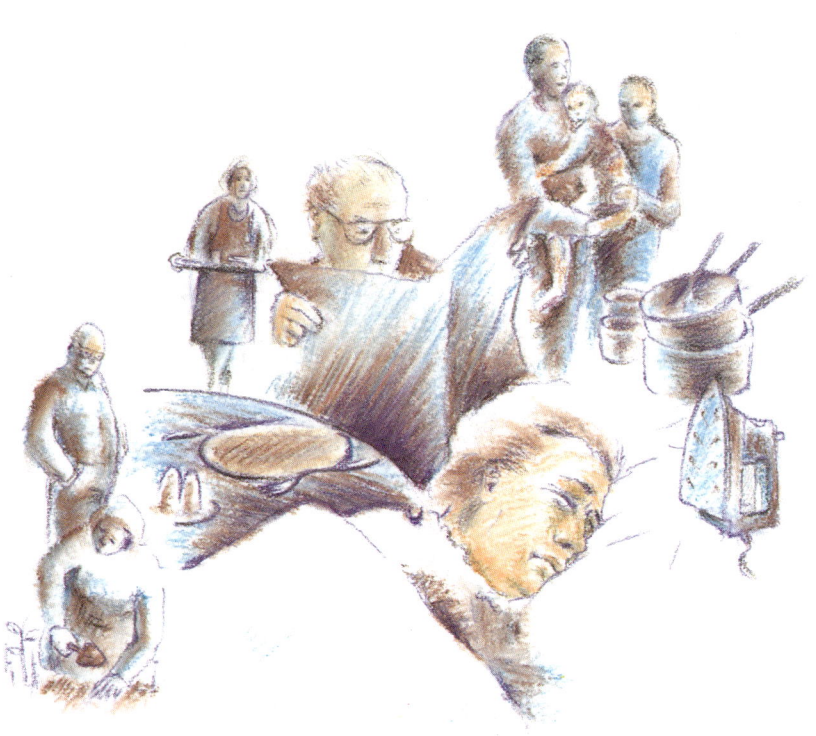

Cheryl – is in her early sixties, and has always lived an active and busy life. But she started to find life increasingly difficult when her husband retired; now she has to cope with his boredom and frustration all day. He has refused to take a part-time job locally, and become demanding and irritable, following her around the house like a young child – if she goes out, he complains about being left alone. Cheryl feels trapped. As a result, she leaves the house less and less often, and in turn resents her loss of freedom and the lack of contact with her friends.

At home Cheryl finds that her husband has no intention of helping her with household chores, and expects her to wait on him as though he was still working; he demands her full attention at all times. Their son lives nearby, and Cheryl had always enjoyed being an active grandmother. But she now finds that she has less and less patience with her grandchildren and has started to put off their visits. Her son and daughter-in-law are upset and concerned, but Cheryl feels that it would be disloyal to explain her problems.

Suffering in silence, Cheryl's resentment with her changed lifestyle has grown and grown. She has become hypercritical and resentful: irritated by what her husband does and bitter about what he does not do. She has become increasingly withdrawn and feels helpless and hopeless. She finds difficulty in sleeping and in settling down to anything; restless and jumpy, she begins numerous tasks, but finishes few.

PERSONAL RELAXATION PROGRAMME
Basic relaxation technique (p56)
Improving posture (p64) and/or Alexander technique (p102)
Homoeopathy (p138) and/or herbalism (p136)
Music (p148) and/or dance therapy (p147)
Art (p150) and/or colour therapy (p142)
Yoga (p110) and/or meditation (p118)
Autogenic therapy (p121) and/or visualization (p122)
Massage (p72) and/or aromatherapy (p80)

STRESS AND RELAXATION

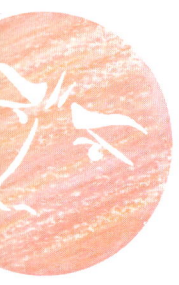

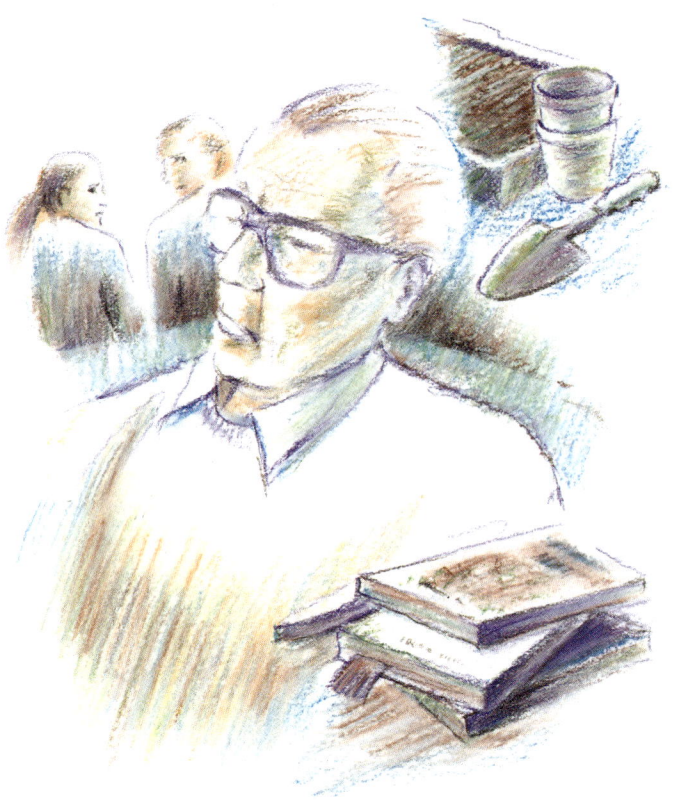

Ian – was forced to retire from work at sixty and is now in his mid sixties. He resents having had to retire early, when he thought that he had many good working years left. At first he enjoyed pottering about the garden that he had always loved, catching up on the backlog of unread books and spending time over the crossword. A widower, he employed a local housewife to help clean the house and prepare his meals.

As time passed, he became more and more bored with his existence. Unfortunately his health, both mental and physical, had started to deteriorate soon after his retirement and he found that he could not concentrate and that even his gardening had developed into an unpleasant chore that caused shortness of breath and a rapid heartbeat. The day after a bout of gardening, he feels stiff, aching and exhausted.

As Ian's feelings of frustration and irritability have grown, he is turning his anger inward; furious at any sign that his mental powers are on the wane, he refuses to attempt anything that might stretch them. His attitude is that if he cannot do a thing well, he will not attempt it.

As he becomes more and more sensitive to the signs of approaching old age, Ian finds that he dreads the noise and disturbance caused by the weekly visits of his young grandchildren. He has little patience with them and they have quickly learnt to keep out of his way. As a result, he has become increasingly cut off from his family and his negative attitude is also losing him friends.

PERSONAL RELAXATION PROGRAMME
Basic relaxation technique (p56)
Music (p148) and art therapy (p150)
Alexander technique (p102)
Acupressure (p84)
Breathing techniques (p60)
Autogenic therapy (p121) and/or autosuggestion (p120)

John – was a fit man in his late sixties. Married and still working as a consultant for his old firm for a few days each week, he would like to continue working all his life. He is physically and mentally fit, too, playing tennis and golf and enjoying walking holidays. He lives a somewhat separate life from his wife, who has always been independent. Recently retired from her career as a lawyer, she now fills her time with bridge games. Both John and his wife feel that they deserve their position in local society and present lifestyle, after the years of juggling jobs and the demands of children.

John's eldest son has recently committed suicide. His wife is inconsolable and John has no idea how to comfort her. Without him realizing it, they have become strangers living under the same roof. Trying to cope not only with his own grief, but also sudden feelings of irrational anger at his son for daring to upset his life and the guilt over his possible neglect of his son during the early years while he strove for success, John has stopped trying to help his wife and withdrawn into his own misery. He still feels distressed by her grief, but is now isolated from both it and her – often wishing that she would just go away.

John now finds it increasingly difficult to go out, convinced that everyone is talking about the suicide. He finds it difficult to concentrate at work and has started to make silly, and possibly dangerous, mistakes – as a result, he has been asked to retire completely. He feels as if all his energy has been sapped by his son's death; he no longer wants to play golf or tennis and has no interest in anything else – he just wants to be left alone. John and his wife are two strangers, wrapped up in their own grief and incapable of helping each other.

PERSONAL RELAXATION PROGRAMME
Basic relaxation technique (p56)
Improving posture (p64)
Music (p148) and/or art therapy (p150)
Yoga (p110) and/or meditation (p118)
Visualization (p122) and/or autosuggestion (p120)
Hydrotherapy (p90)

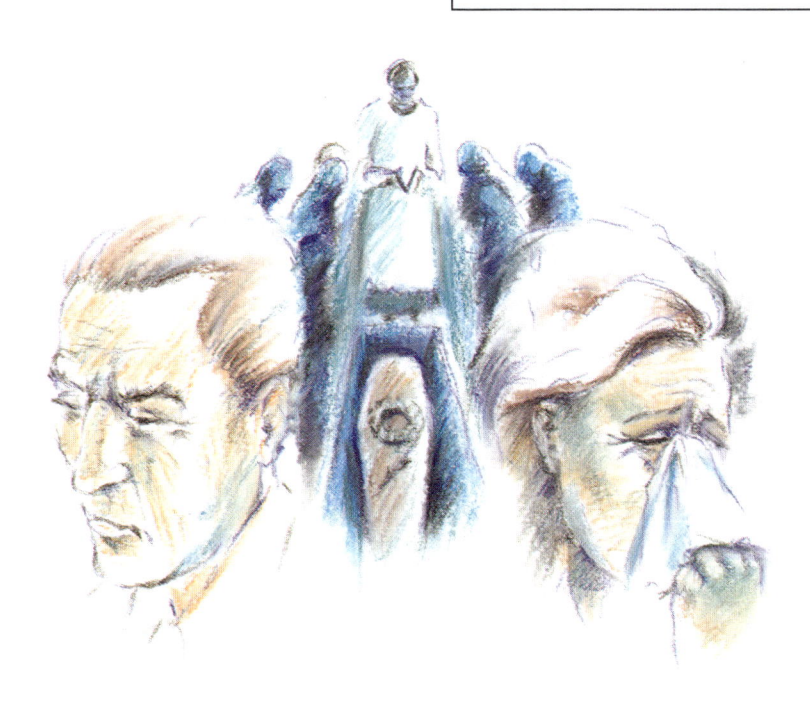

SYMPTOM AND THERAPY FLOW CHARTS

Use these flow charts as a way of starting to treat your stress symptoms and increasing relaxation. All the therapies described in this book help to reduce stress and promote relaxation to a certain extent, but some techniques are more effective than others when it comes to dealing with particular types, or particular symptoms, of stress. So the charts that follow provide a useful guide to what symptoms tend to be associated with what problems, and what therapies can be used to relieve the symptoms and treat the problems. However, stress and relaxation are complex and interrelated phenomena, so the charts should only be treated as a guide: a starting point on your own personal journey through the possibilities available. If the recommended treatment is not working as well as you think it should, try others, until you find the right therapy for you.

ACHES & PAINS

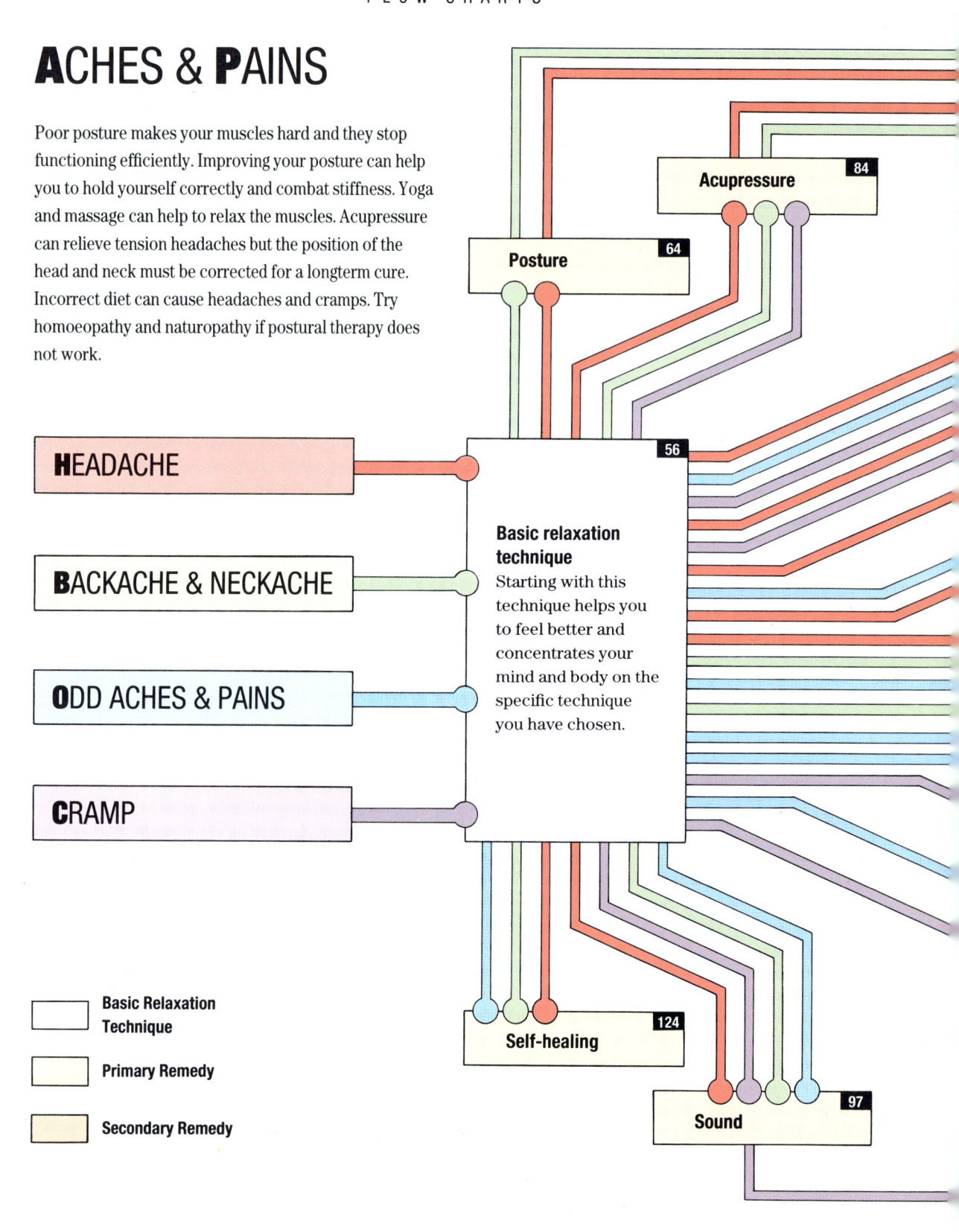

Poor posture makes your muscles hard and they stop functioning efficiently. Improving your posture can help you to hold yourself correctly and combat stiffness. Yoga and massage can help to relax the muscles. Acupressure can relieve tension headaches but the position of the head and neck must be corrected for a longterm cure. Incorrect diet can cause headaches and cramps. Try homoeopathy and naturopathy if postural therapy does not work.

HEADACHE

BACKACHE & NECKACHE

ODD ACHES & PAINS

CRAMP

Acupressure 84

Posture 64

Basic relaxation technique 56
Starting with this technique helps you to feel better and concentrates your mind and body on the specific technique you have chosen.

Self-healing 124

Sound 97

Basic Relaxation Technique

Primary Remedy

Secondary Remedy

ACHES & PAINS

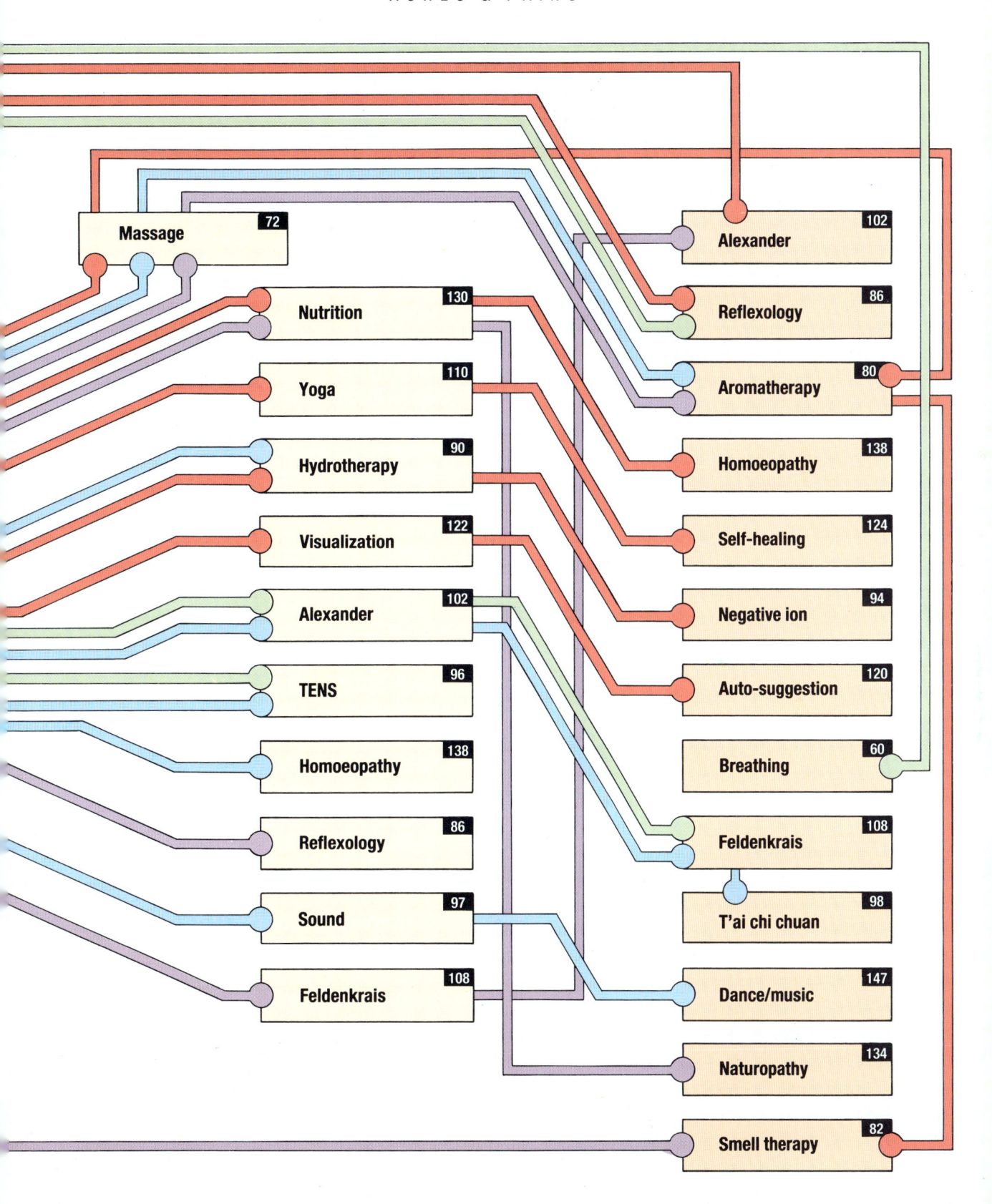

Therapy	Page
Massage	72
Nutrition	130
Yoga	110
Hydrotherapy	90
Visualization	122
Alexander	102
TENS	96
Homoeopathy	138
Reflexology	86
Sound	97
Feldenkrais	108
Alexander	102
Reflexology	86
Aromatherapy	80
Homoeopathy	138
Self-healing	124
Negative ion	94
Auto-suggestion	120
Breathing	60
Feldenkrais	108
T'ai chi chuan	98
Dance/music	147
Naturopathy	134
Smell therapy	82

39

/ FLOW CHARTS

DIGESTIVE PROBLEMS

Problems with the digestive tract are often the result of anxiety and stress. Some of the techniques suggested below, such as visualization, self-hypnosis, meditation, music and art, encourage peace and mental relaxation. Digestive tract problems can also result from bad diet or a food allergy, so consider naturopathy, nutritional medicine or herbalism. Yoga has a dual effect: it not only helps to relax and calm, but also has a beneficial effect on the internal organs of the body.

Yoga 110

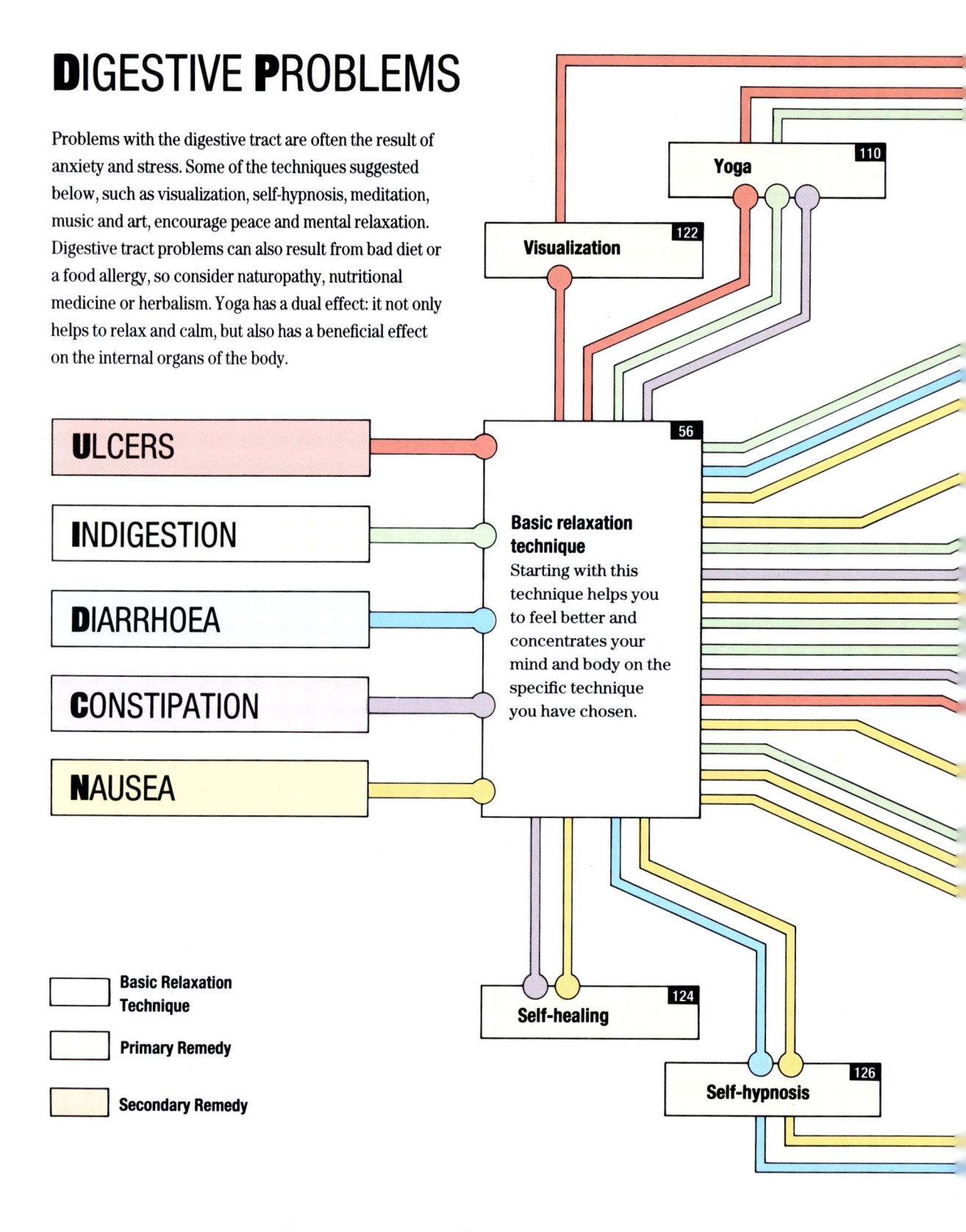

Visualization 122

ULCERS

INDIGESTION

DIARRHOEA

CONSTIPATION

NAUSEA

Basic relaxation technique 56
Starting with this technique helps you to feel better and concentrates your mind and body on the specific technique you have chosen.

Self-healing 124

Self-hypnosis 126

☐ Basic Relaxation Technique

☐ Primary Remedy

☐ Secondary Remedy

DIGESTIVE PROBLEMS

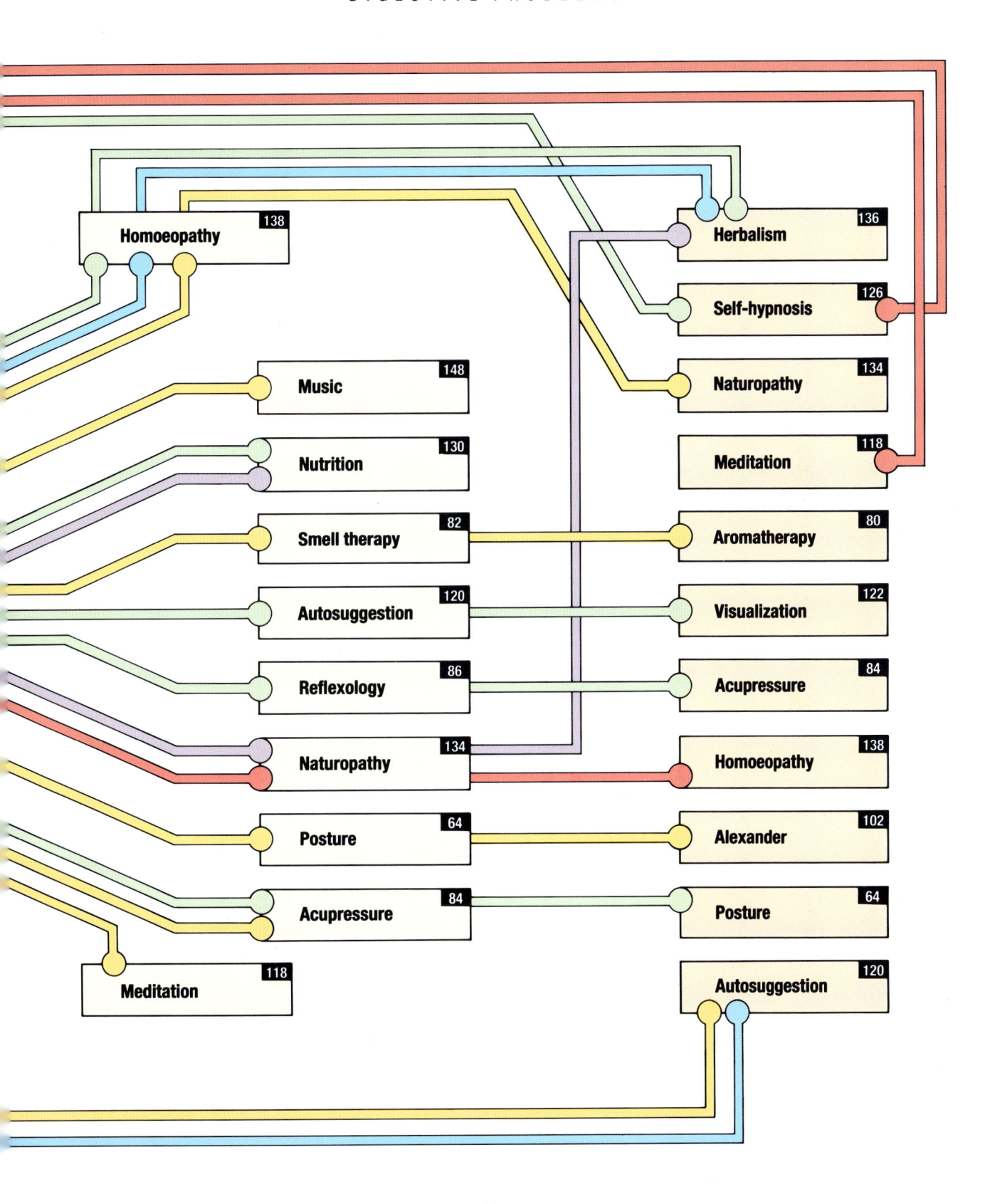

Homoeopathy 138	Herbalism 136
Music 148	Self-hypnosis 126
Nutrition 130	Naturopathy 134
Smell therapy 82	Meditation 118
Autosuggestion 120	Aromatherapy 80
Reflexology 86	Visualization 122
Naturopathy 134	Acupressure 84
Posture 64	Homoeopathy 138
Acupressure 84	Alexander 102
Meditation 118	Posture 64
	Autosuggestion 120

41

PALPITATIONS

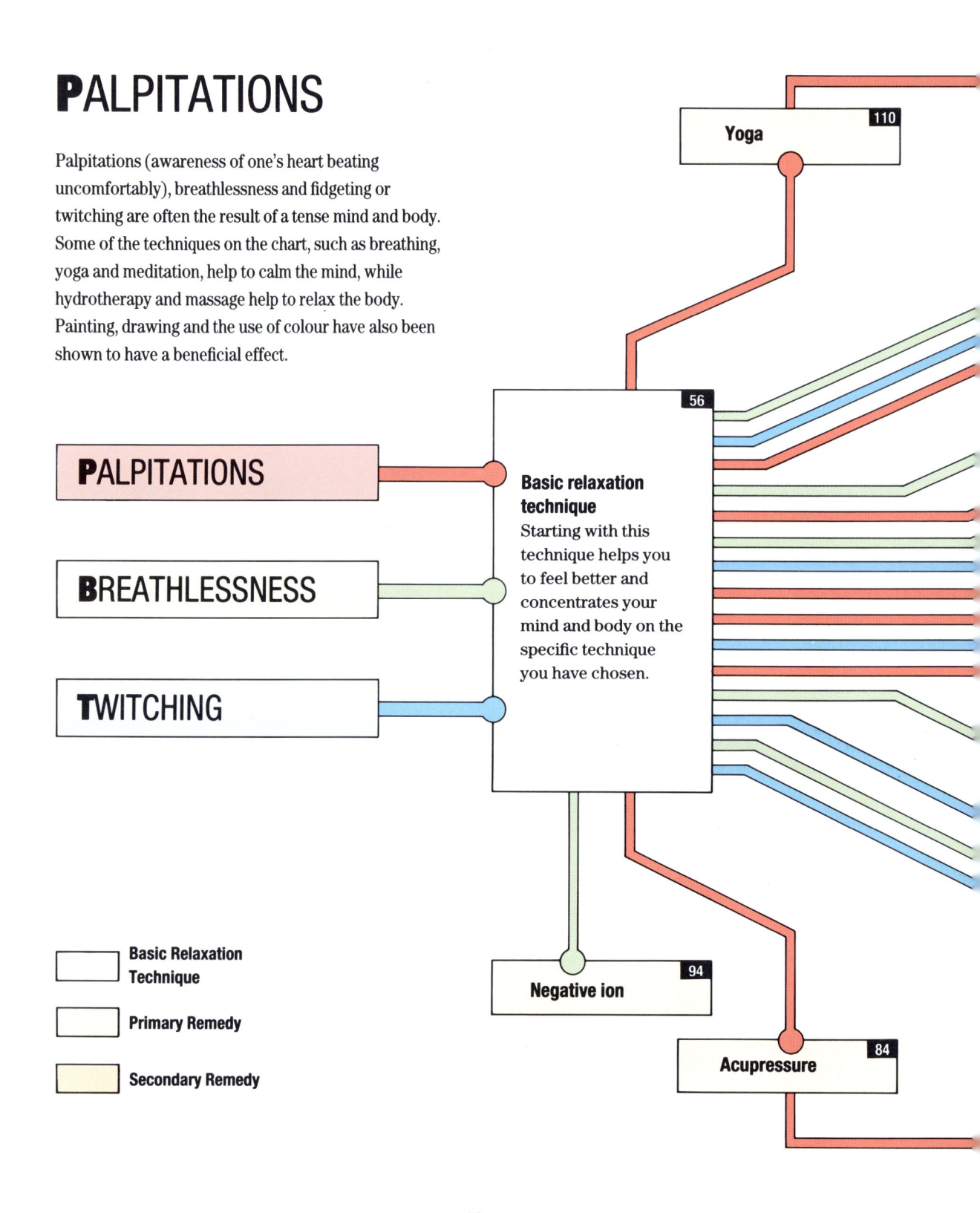

Palpitations (awareness of one's heart beating uncomfortably), breathlessness and fidgeting or twitching are often the result of a tense mind and body. Some of the techniques on the chart, such as breathing, yoga and meditation, help to calm the mind, while hydrotherapy and massage help to relax the body. Painting, drawing and the use of colour have also been shown to have a beneficial effect.

PALPITATIONS

BREATHLESSNESS

TWITCHING

Basic Relaxation Technique

Primary Remedy

Secondary Remedy

Yoga 110

Basic relaxation technique 56
Starting with this technique helps you to feel better and concentrates your mind and body on the specific technique you have chosen.

Negative ion 94

Acupressure 84

PALPITATIONS

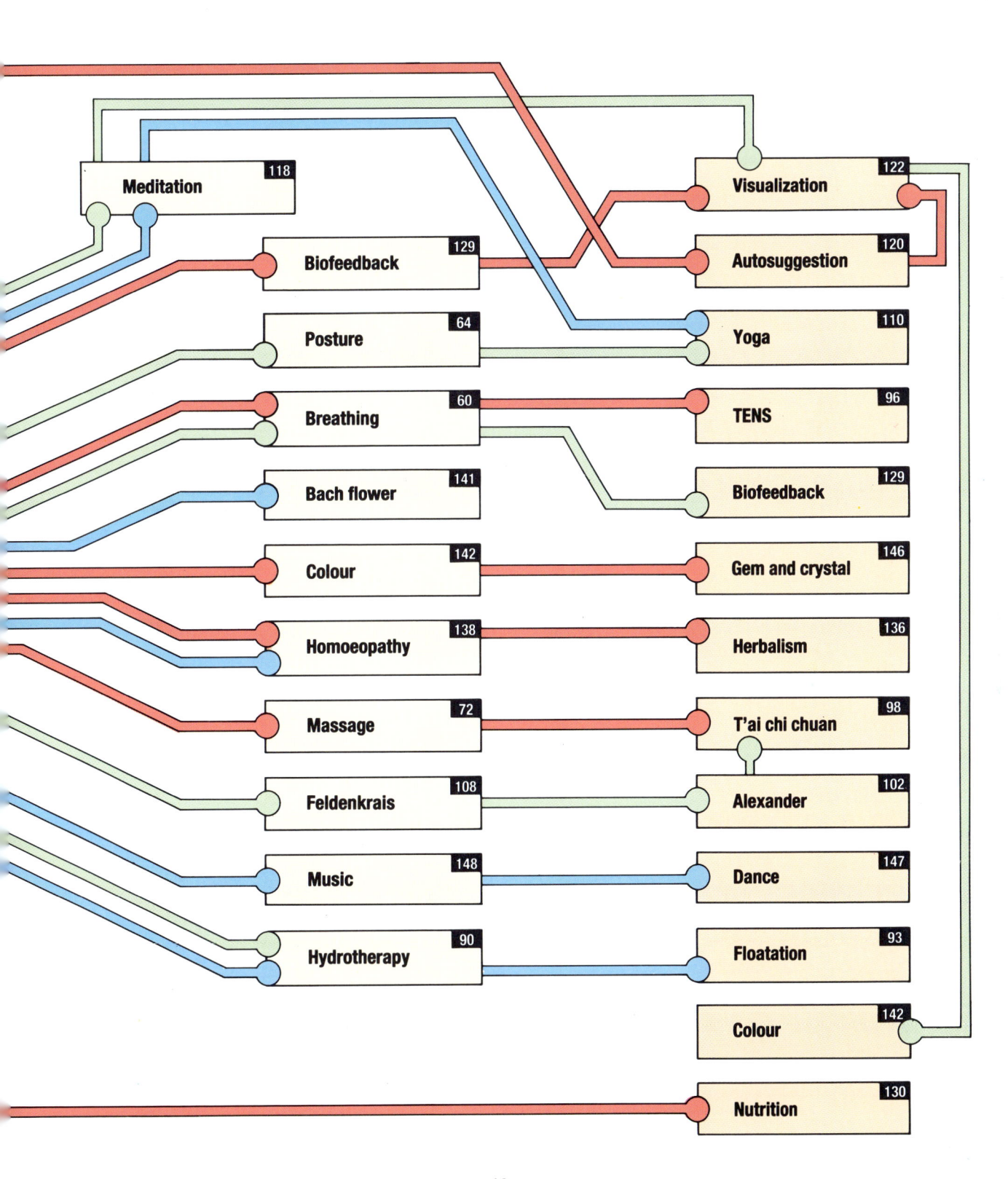

Meditation 118	Visualization 122
Biofeedback 129	Autosuggestion 120
Posture 64	Yoga 110
Breathing 60	TENS 96
Bach flower 141	Biofeedback 129
Colour 142	Gem and crystal 146
Homoeopathy 138	Herbalism 136
Massage 72	T'ai chi chuan 98
Feldenkrais 108	Alexander 102
Music 148	Dance 147
Hydrotherapy 90	Floatation 93
	Colour 142
	Nutrition 130

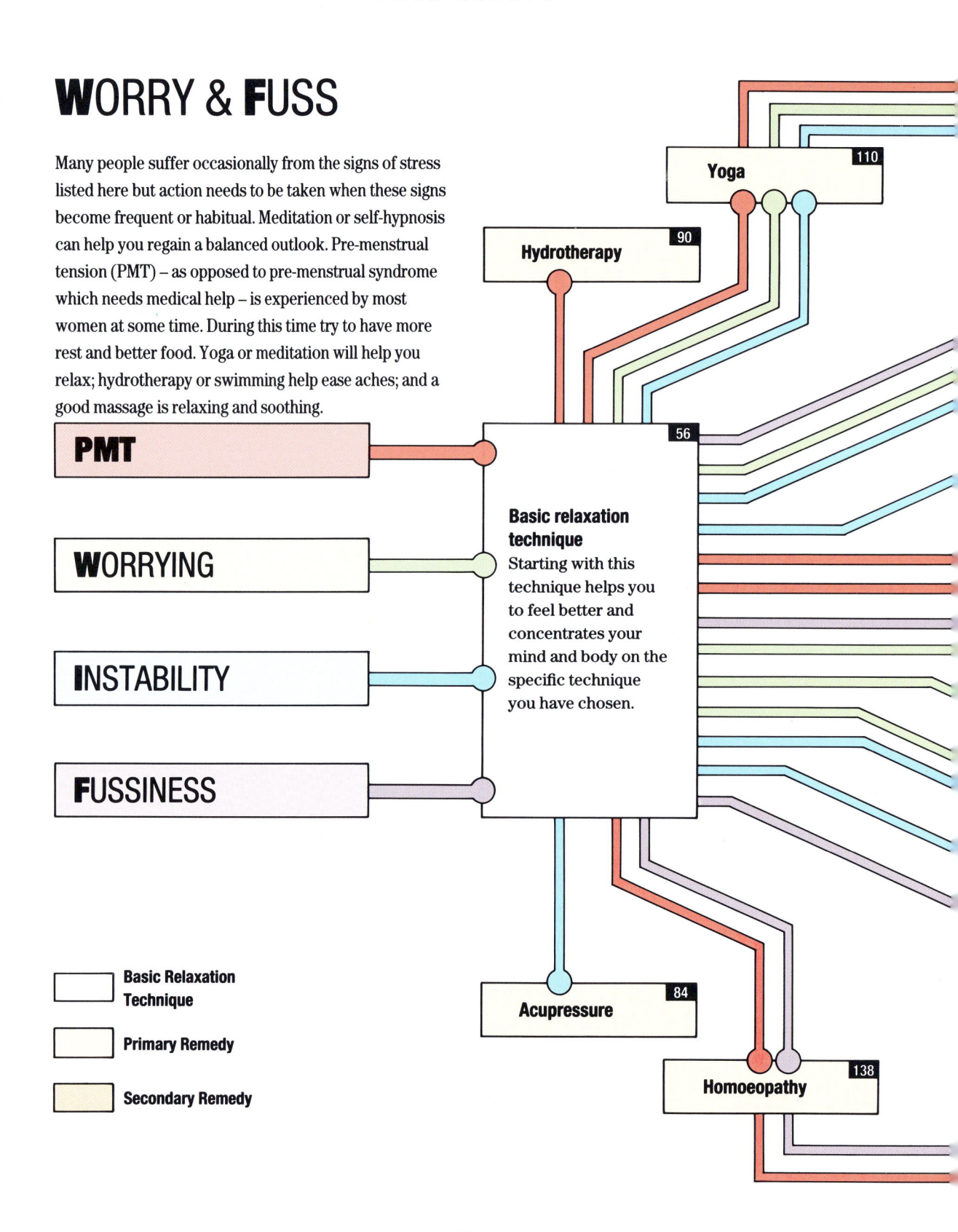

FLOW CHARTS

WORRY & FUSS

Many people suffer occasionally from the signs of stress listed here but action needs to be taken when these signs become frequent or habitual. Meditation or self-hypnosis can help you regain a balanced outlook. Pre-menstrual tension (PMT) – as opposed to pre-menstrual syndrome which needs medical help – is experienced by most women at some time. During this time try to have more rest and better food. Yoga or meditation will help you relax; hydrotherapy or swimming help ease aches; and a good massage is relaxing and soothing.

PMT

WORRYING

INSTABILITY

FUSSINESS

Yoga 110

Hydrotherapy 90

Basic relaxation technique 56
Starting with this technique helps you to feel better and concentrates your mind and body on the specific technique you have chosen.

Acupressure 84

Homoeopathy 138

Basic Relaxation Technique

Primary Remedy

Secondary Remedy

44

WORRY & FUSS

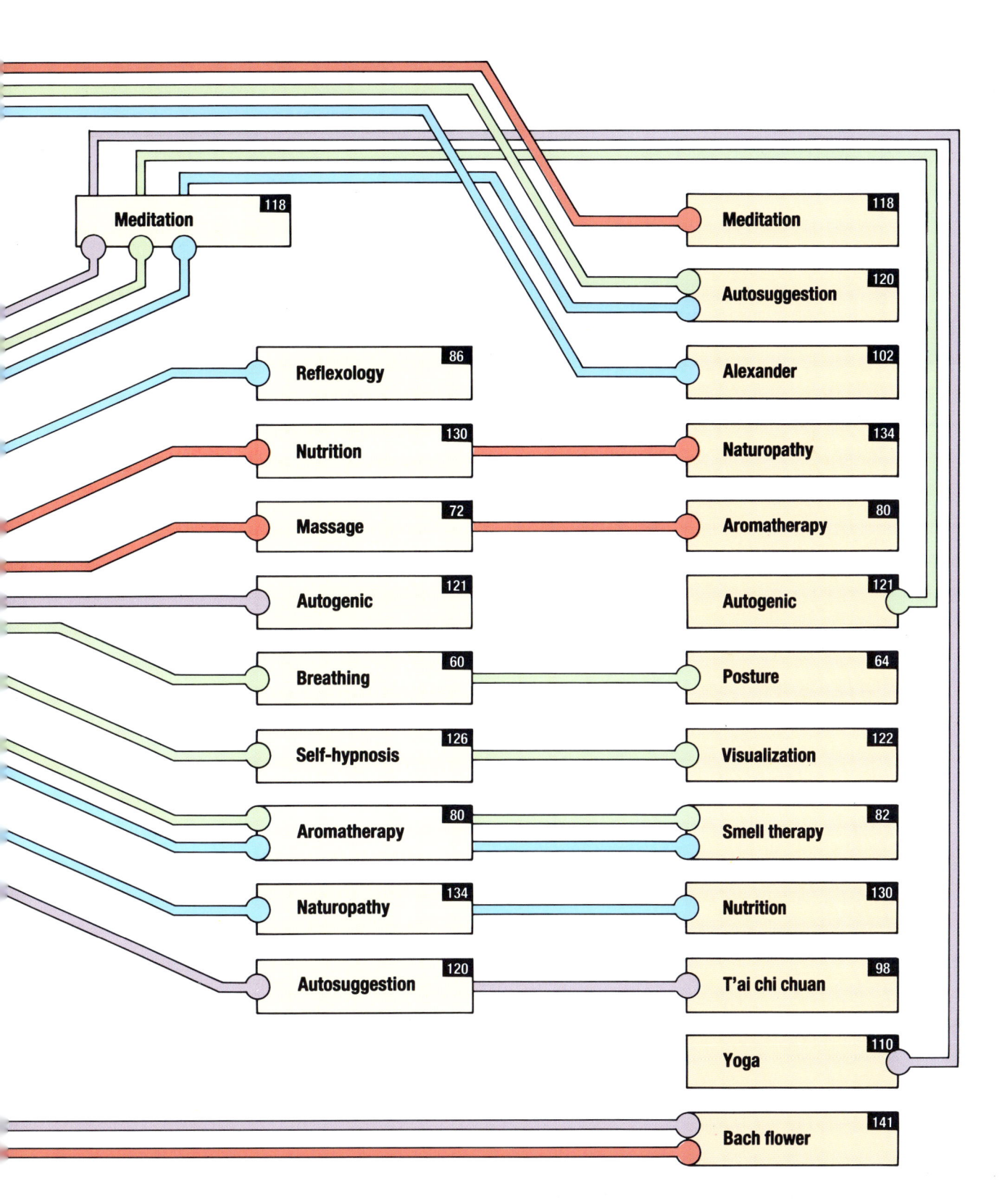

Meditation	118

Meditation	118
Autosuggestion	120
Alexander	102
Naturopathy	134
Aromatherapy	80
Autogenic	121
Posture	64
Visualization	122
Smell therapy	82
Nutrition	130
T'ai chi chuan	98
Yoga	110
Bach flower	141

Reflexology	86
Nutrition	130
Massage	72
Autogenic	121
Breathing	60
Self-hypnosis	126
Aromatherapy	80
Naturopathy	134
Autosuggestion	120

45

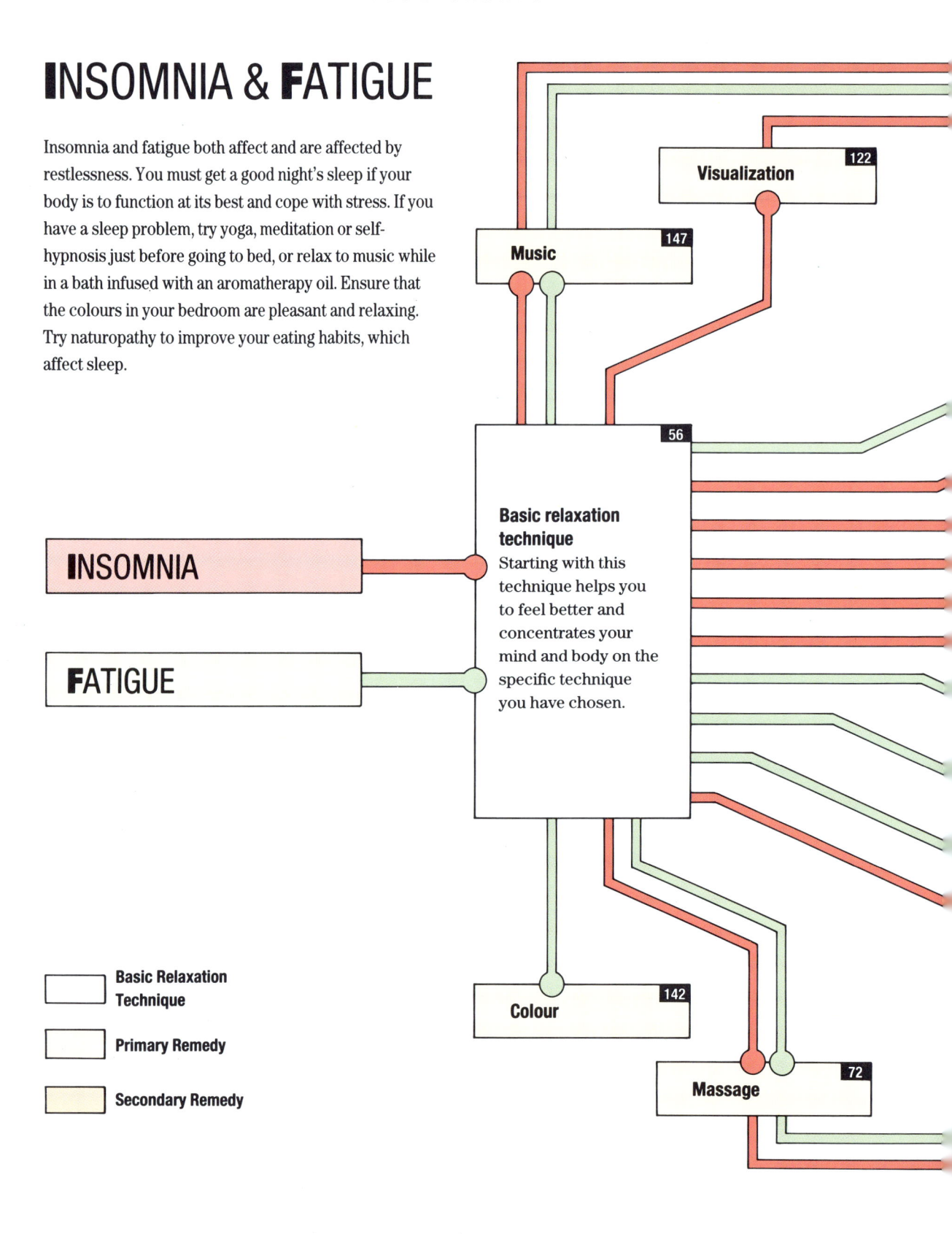

FLOW CHARTS

INSOMNIA & FATIGUE

Insomnia and fatigue both affect and are affected by restlessness. You must get a good night's sleep if your body is to function at its best and cope with stress. If you have a sleep problem, try yoga, meditation or self-hypnosis just before going to bed, or relax to music while in a bath infused with an aromatherapy oil. Ensure that the colours in your bedroom are pleasant and relaxing. Try naturopathy to improve your eating habits, which affect sleep.

Visualization 122

Music 147

INSOMNIA

FATIGUE

Basic relaxation technique 56
Starting with this technique helps you to feel better and concentrates your mind and body on the specific technique you have chosen.

Colour 142

Massage 72

Basic Relaxation Technique

Primary Remedy

Secondary Remedy

INSOMNIA & FATIGUE

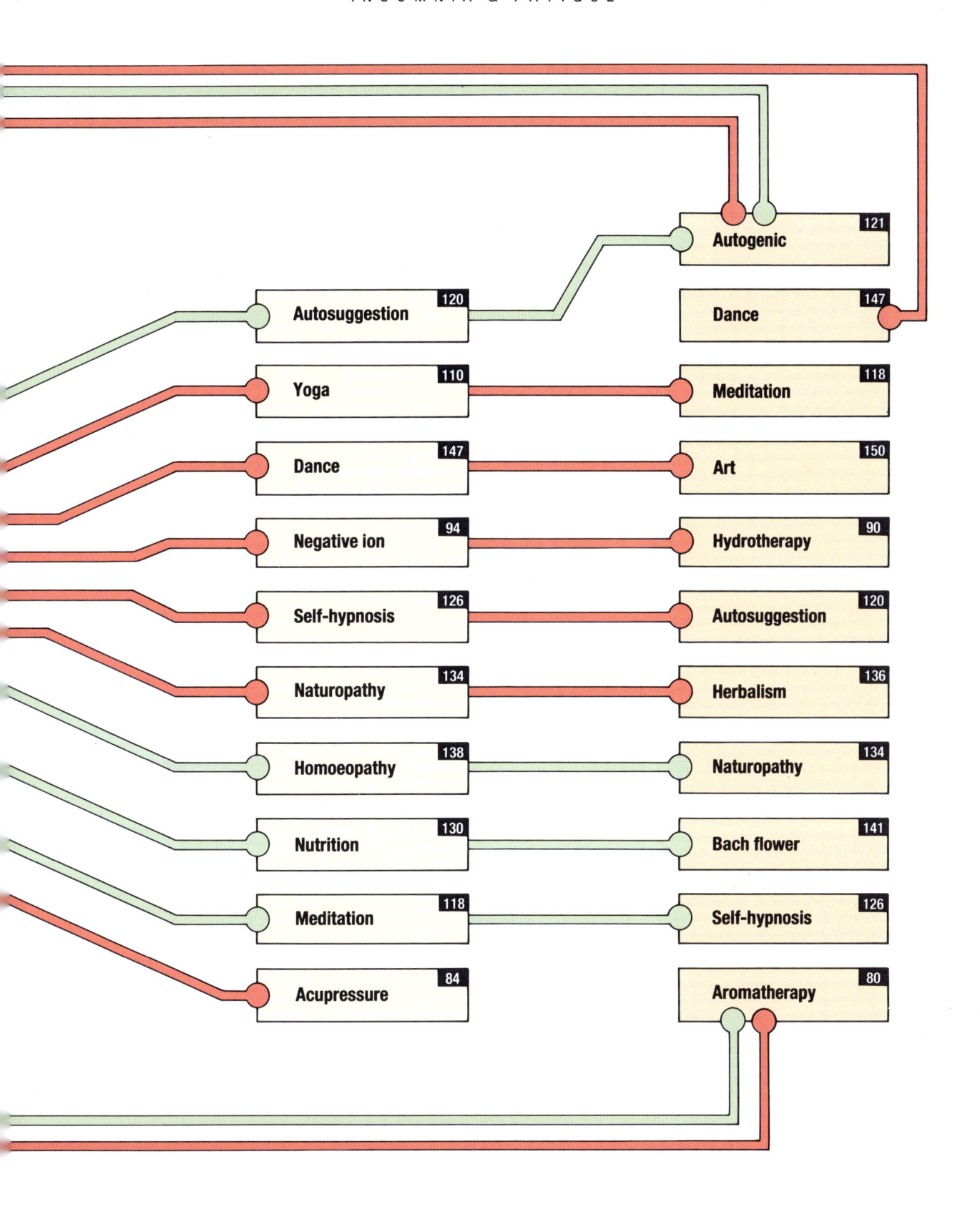

Autosuggestion 120	Autogenic 121
Yoga 110	Dance 147
Dance 147	Meditation 118
Negative ion 94	Art 150
Self-hypnosis 126	Hydrotherapy 90
Naturopathy 134	Autosuggestion 120
Homoeopathy 138	Herbalism 136
Nutrition 130	Naturopathy 134
Meditation 118	Bach flower 141
Acupressure 84	Self-hypnosis 126
	Aromatherapy 80

FLOW CHARTS

Hidden Problems

Refusing to admit the existence of a problem can cause the signs of stress listed below. They are all caused by a person running away from problems that are causing stress, rather than confronting them and coping with them. Relaxation techniques help to combat this tendency, by giving you the insight, will-power and ability to deal with problems as they occur. At the same time, techniques such as naturopathy and homoeopathy can help to combat the damage being done to your body by, for example, excessive smoking and drinking.

- **S**MOKING
- **D**RINKING
- **O**VER **E**ATING
- **C**ASUAL **S**EX
- **L**OSS OF **L**IBIDO

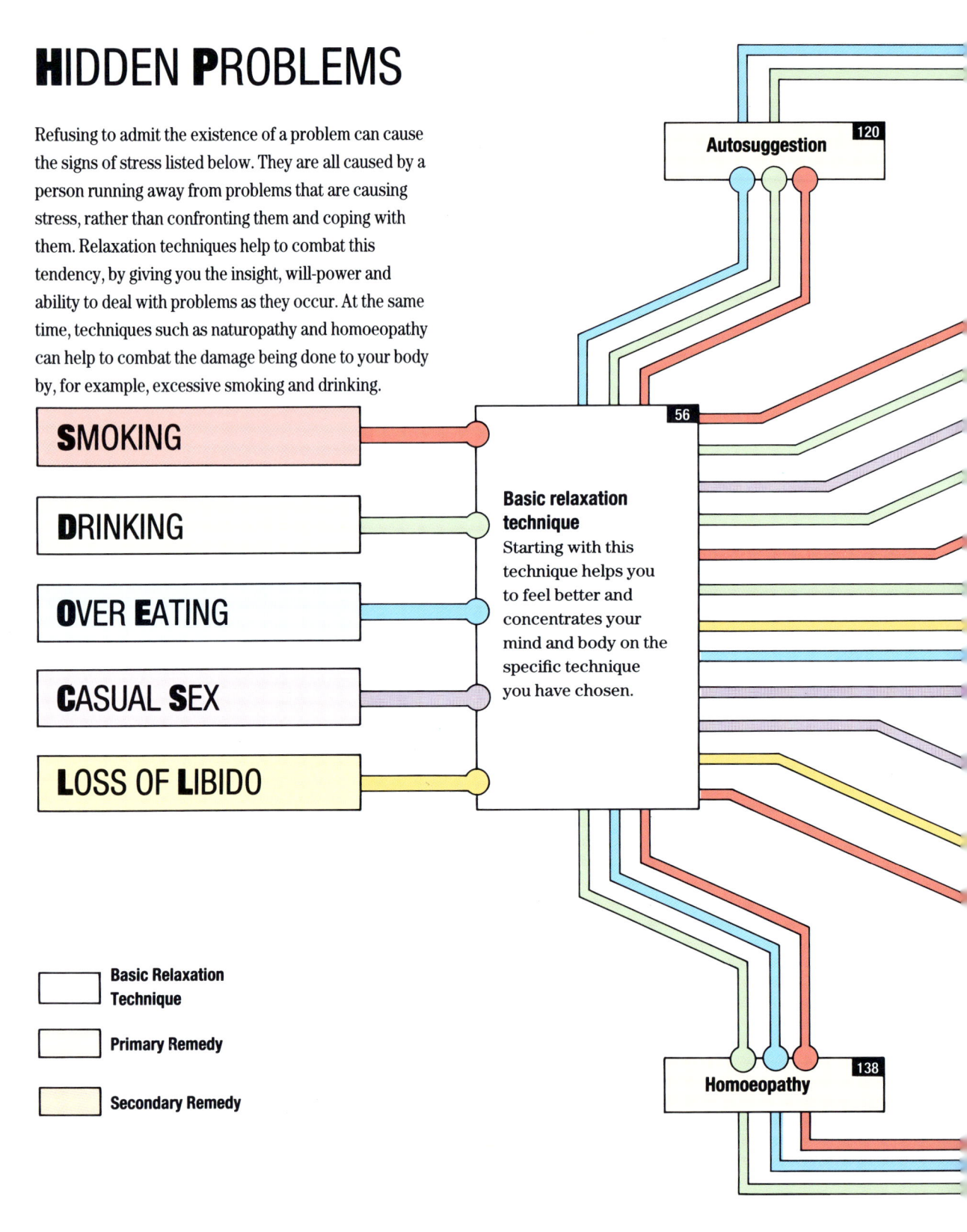

Autosuggestion 120

Basic relaxation technique 56
Starting with this technique helps you to feel better and concentrates your mind and body on the specific technique you have chosen.

Homoeopathy 138

- Basic Relaxation Technique
- Primary Remedy
- Secondary Remedy

HIDDEN PROBLEMS

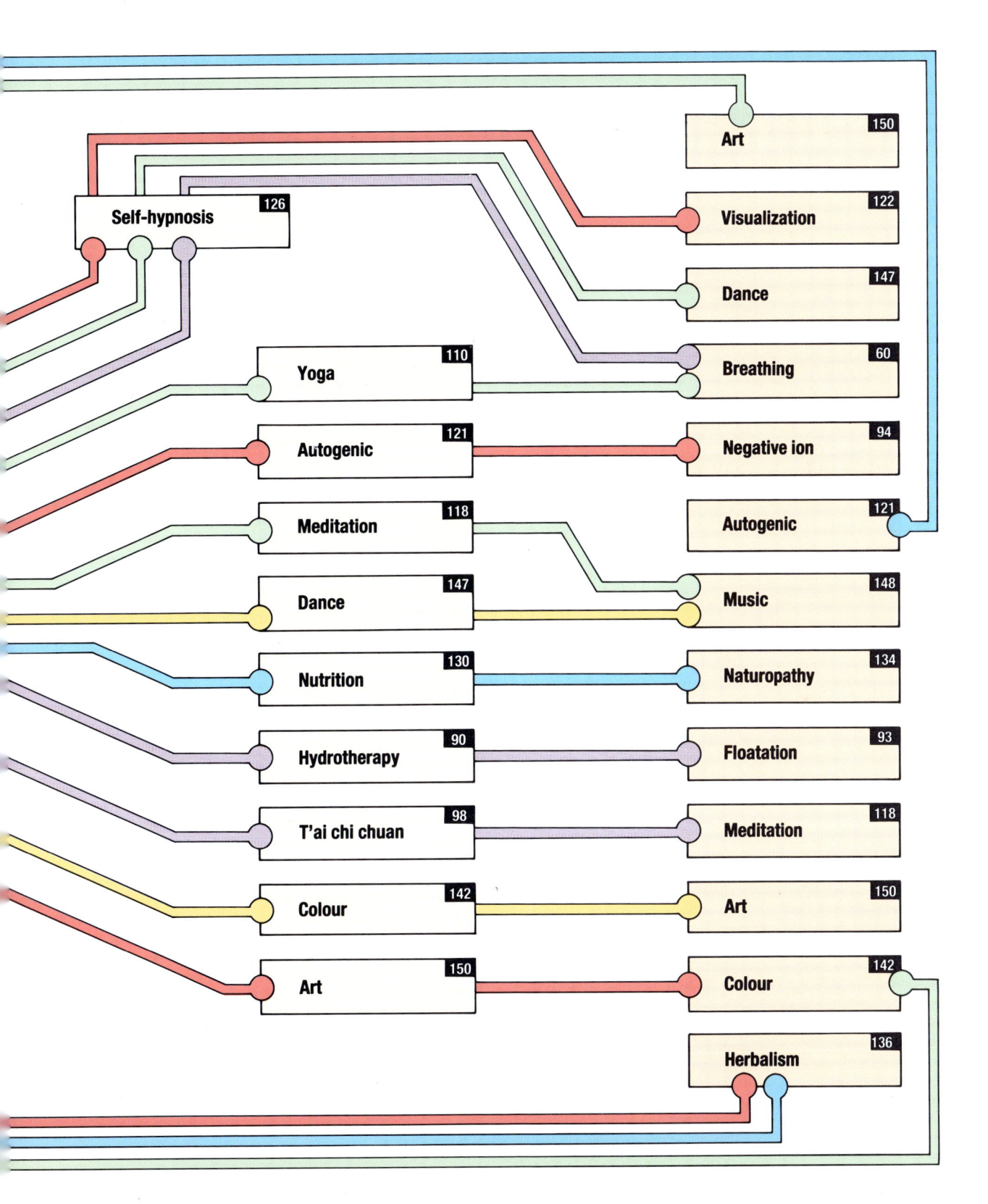

Box	Page
Art	150
Self-hypnosis	126
Visualization	122
Dance	147
Yoga	110
Breathing	60
Autogenic	121
Negative ion	94
Meditation	118
Autogenic	121
Dance	147
Music	148
Nutrition	130
Naturopathy	134
Hydrotherapy	90
Floatation	93
T'ai chi chuan	98
Meditation	118
Colour	142
Art	150
Art	150
Colour	142
Herbalism	136

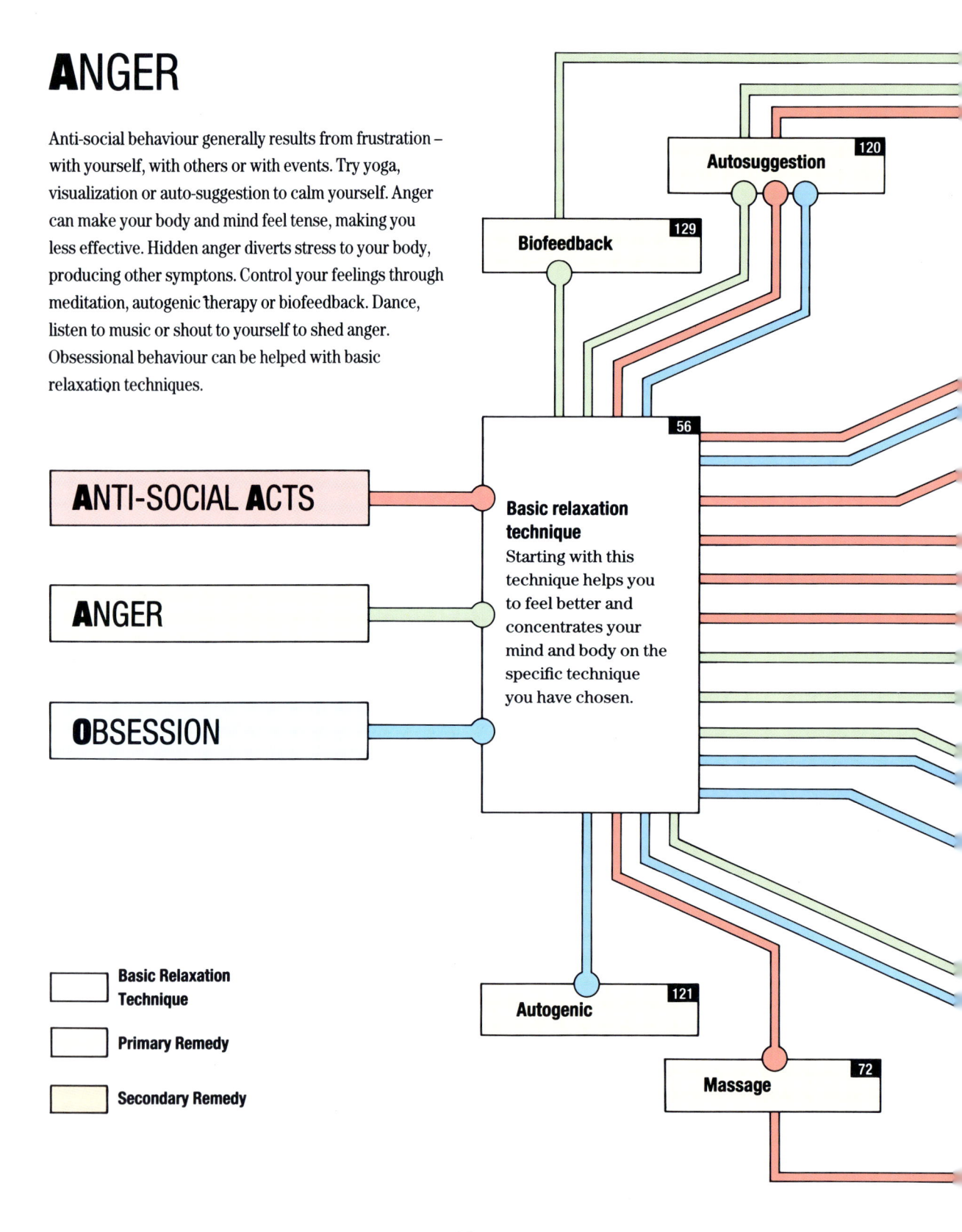

FLOW CHARTS

ANGER

Anti-social behaviour generally results from frustration – with yourself, with others or with events. Try yoga, visualization or auto-suggestion to calm yourself. Anger can make your body and mind feel tense, making you less effective. Hidden anger diverts stress to your body, producing other symptons. Control your feelings through meditation, autogenic therapy or biofeedback. Dance, listen to music or shout to yourself to shed anger. Obsessional behaviour can be helped with basic relaxation techniques.

ANTI-SOCIAL **A**CTS

ANGER

OBSESSION

- Basic Relaxation Technique
- Primary Remedy
- Secondary Remedy

Autosuggestion 120

Biofeedback 129

Basic relaxation technique 56
Starting with this technique helps you to feel better and concentrates your mind and body on the specific technique you have chosen.

Autogenic 121

Massage 72

50

ANGER

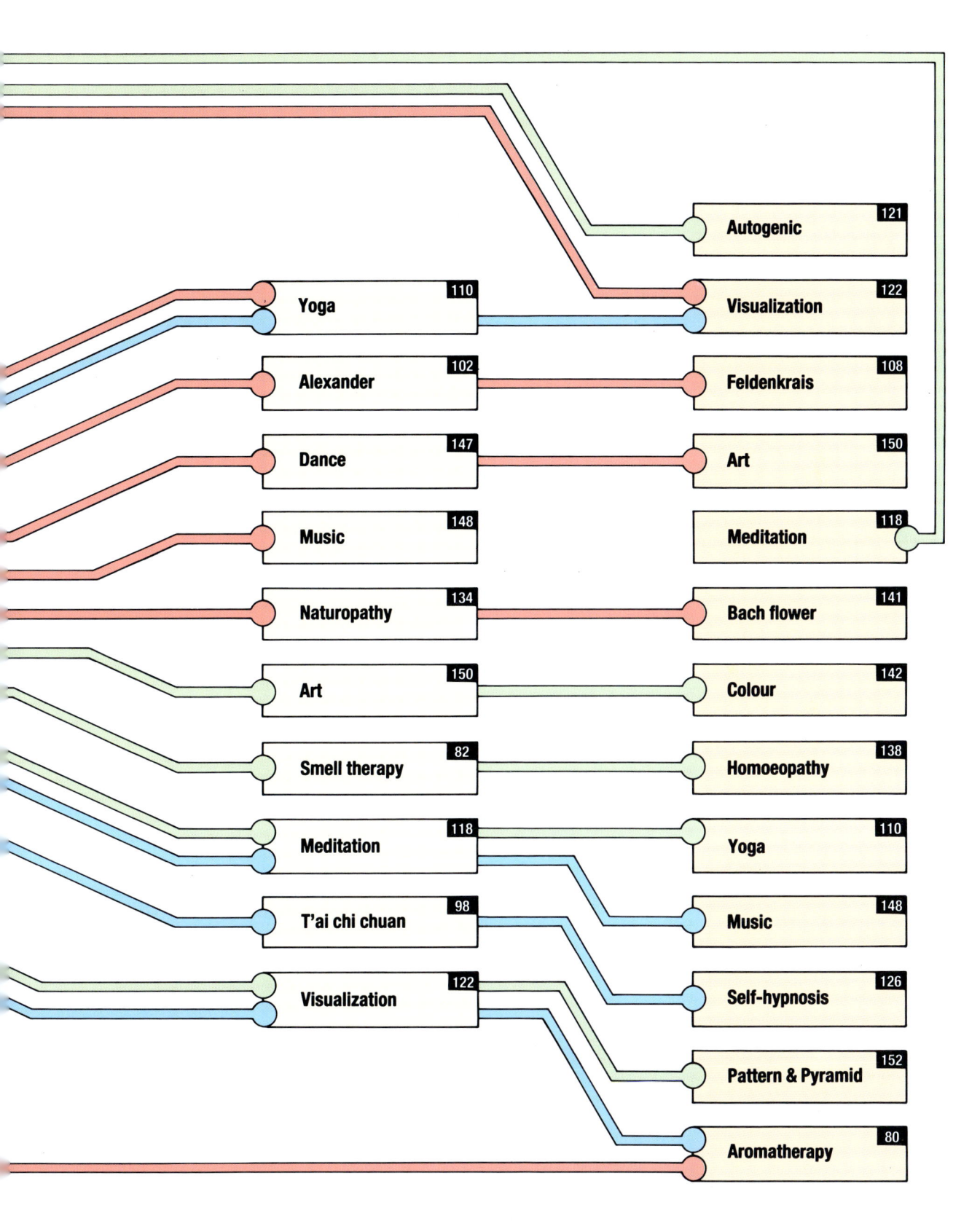

Therapy	Page
Autogenic	121
Yoga	110
Visualization	122
Alexander	102
Feldenkrais	108
Dance	147
Art	150
Music	148
Meditation	118
Naturopathy	134
Bach flower	141
Art	150
Colour	142
Smell therapy	82
Homoeopathy	138
Meditation	118
Yoga	110
T'ai chi chuan	98
Music	148
Visualization	122
Self-hypnosis	126
Pattern & Pyramid	152
Aromatherapy	80

FLOW CHARTS

DEPRESSION

Everyone feels tense and depressed at certain times in their life. To help you relax during one of these periods, try one of the mental techniques, such as meditation, yoga or autogenic therapy. Listen to soothing music to relieve tension or cheerful, lively music if you feel miserable. A good massage with an aromatherapy oil will help to relieve tension and ease depression, as will hydrotherapy. People are inclined to hold themselves badly when they feel depressed or tense, so think about improving your posture.

Colour 142

Art 150

DEPRESSION

TENSION & ANXIETY

Basic relaxation technique 56
Starting with this technique helps you to feel better and concentrates your mind and body on the specific technique you have chosen.

Massage 72

Hydrotherapy 90

☐ Basic Relaxation Technique

☐ Primary Remedy

☐ Secondary Remedy

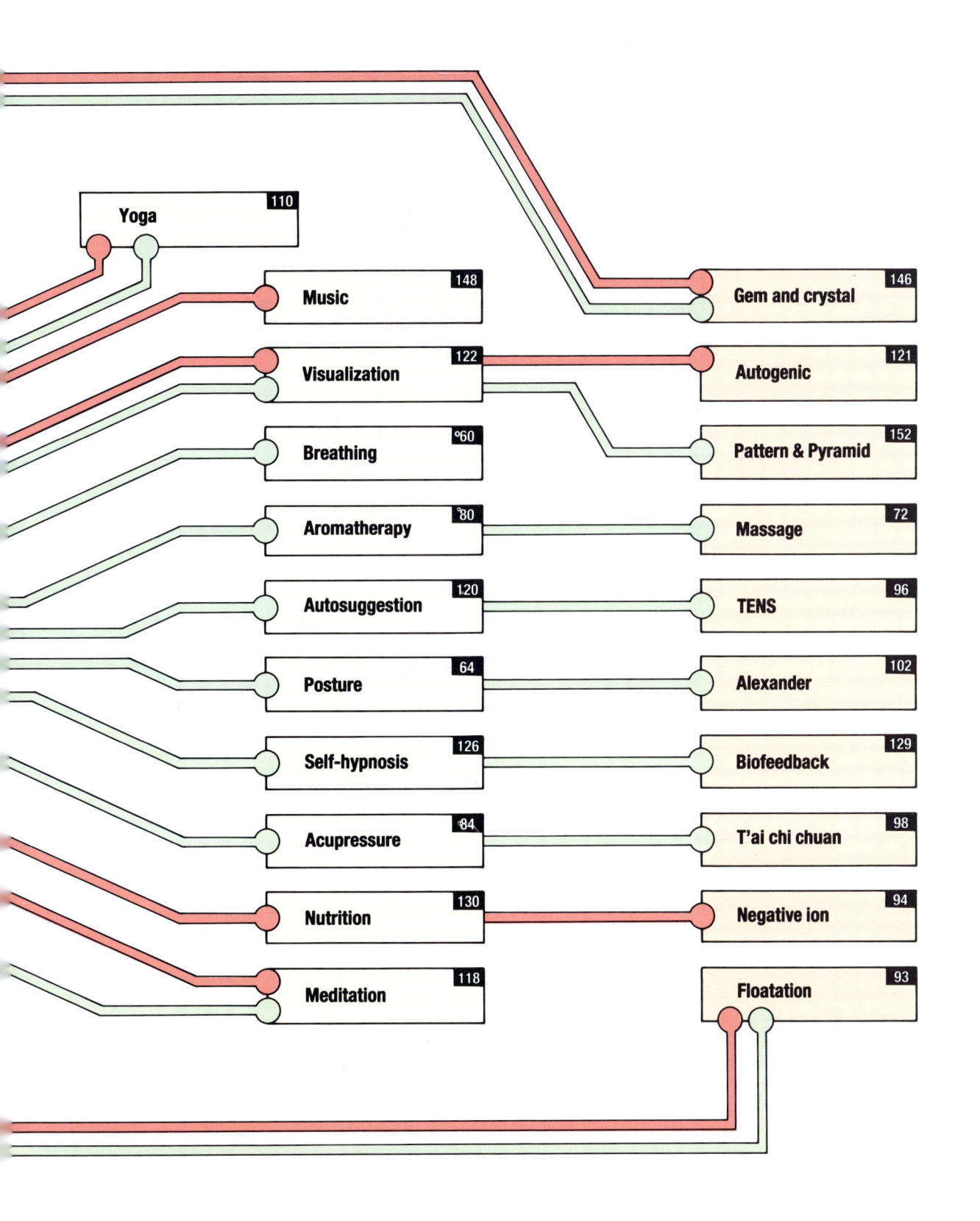

DEPRESSION

	Page		Page
Yoga	110		
Music	148	Gem and crystal	146
Visualization	122	Autogenic	121
Breathing	60	Pattern & Pyramid	152
Aromatherapy	80	Massage	72
Autosuggestion	120	TENS	96
Posture	64	Alexander	102
Self-hypnosis	126	Biofeedback	129
Acupressure	84	T'ai chi chuan	98
Nutrition	130	Negative ion	94
Meditation	118	Floatation	93

BASIC RELAXATION TECHNIQUES

This section covers techniques which can be used on their own or as a prelude to all the general techniques in the book. For example, it is good to do a Basic Relaxation routine before you start any of the techniques. Breathing properly is a very important part of feeling good and staying healthy, and simply becoming aware of how to breathe properly is a good start in this direction. Good posture is fundamental – not only does it help you breathe properly, but it is an instant pick-me-up and makes you look and feel better – which in turn makes other people respond to you better. Another quick relaxation technique is to do warming and stretching exercises (which are also important for the more physical techniques in the next section as it is essential to warm your muscles before any form of exercise). The stretches can be done first thing in the morning to energize you, in the evening to relax you, or at any time of day if you have been sitting still for a long time and need to unlock your muscles.

BASIC RELAXATION TECHNIQUE

A self-help technique to reduce accumulated stress in the body, by progressively contracting and relaxing the muscle groups that store tension. While it is essential that our muscles maintain a certain amount of tension to support posture and movement, it is when our bodies have to move unnaturally or under stress that the result can be extra, unnecessary tension in certain muscles – for example in the neck and shoulders. This itself causes symptoms of stress – headaches, aches and pains and general tiredness, for example – and so the vicious circle is established.

To break out of this circle, we need to know how to release excess tension from the muscles – this is the first step in relaxation, and is used in all the various techniques. To succeed, however, one important lesson should be borne in mind: that is, a recognition that most of the time we tend to concentrate on what is happening in the outside world around us, whereas the essence of relaxation is to bring that focus back inside ourselves, so that we may become sensitive to the tensions within and begin to relieve them.

Method

Put on loose, comfortable clothes, making sure that your feet are warm.

1 Lie down in a quiet, warm, dark room, using either the floor, a mat or a firm bed – this is perhaps the best position for a beginner, though alternative positions are given below. Place a pillow or cushion under your head and knees. Either let your hands and arms rest by your side or gently upon your stomach, whichever feels the most comfortable.

2 Check that you feel really comfortable. If necessary use more pillows – perhaps under your feet and forearms. Only start the technique once you are certain of your comfort.

3 Relax and let your mind go blank. Take a couple of deep breaths and sigh the air away.

4 Now you are ready to start reducing tension in your muscles. The technique involves 'letting go' of all the muscles in the body, starting at the toes, working gradually up the body and ending with the face. To begin, concentrate on your left foot. Tense all the muscles – curling the toes and scrunching the foot. Hold for a few seconds. Let go, and make them feel floppy, heavy and warm, as if they are sinking into the pillow. It may take a little practice to perfect this technique, but it will come if you persevere.

Relax your knees

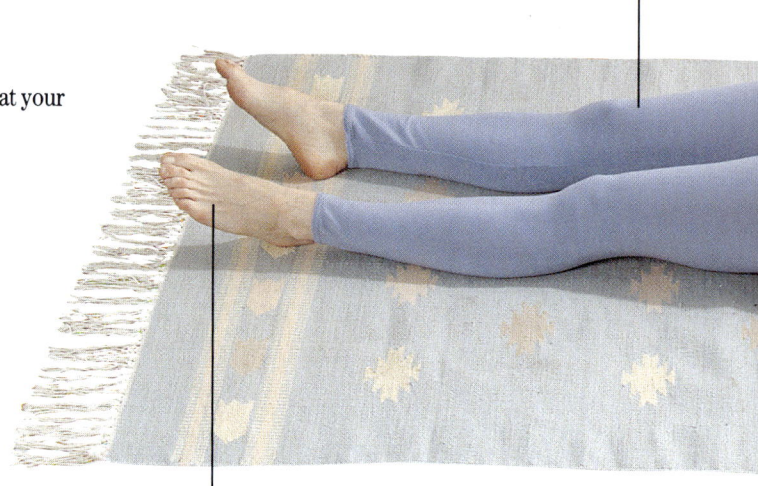

Allow your feet to fall outwards

BASIC RELAXATION TECHNIQUE

5 Move on to the calf muscles of the left leg. Tense the muscles, hold and let go. Feel the heaviness and warmth of the leg and foot.

6 Apply the same technique to the left thigh. Concentrate on the left leg – does it feel heavy, warm, and relaxed? Is it sinking into the floor or bed? If the answers are 'no', tense the whole leg, hold it in tension until it feels difficult to hold the position any longer, then let go completely.

7 Repeat the same process with the right leg.

8 When both legs feel heavy and numb, continue moving up the body. Clench your buttocks tightly and let go; pull in your stomach muscles, hold tight, relax – let them fall back towards the spine, into the floor or bed. Feel the warmth spreading up your body.

9 Breathe deeply and evenly a few times, then sigh the breath away – imagine you are sighing all the tension out of your body.

10 Move on to your left hand, squeeze your hand into a fist, hold tight and let go. Tighten the muscles in the arm, let them flop. Continue with your right arm. Repeat if the arms are not relaxed and heavy. They should feel numb and impossible to move.

11 Hunch your shoulders up towards your ears, hold, let go; let them sink into the floor. It may be necessary to repeat this movement a few times as we hold a lot of tension in our shoulders. Pull the shoulders up towards the ceiling and let them flop back into the ground. Repeat a couple of times.

12 Rock your head gently from side to side in order to loosen the neck. Feel the total relaxation of the body, breathe deeply a few times. Relax, feel the warmth and quiet.

13 The face is the most difficult part of the body to relax: yawn widely with an open mouth, let go; purse the lips out in a pout, then relax; frown fiercely, let go; move the scalp by raising the eyebrows, then relax.

14 The whole body should now be relaxed. Breathe evenly in and out, saying to yourself with each breath that you feel more and more relaxed, peaceful and warm.

15 Rest, relaxed and warm for around 15 minutes. Do not jump up and start racing around. Let yourself come to slowly and gently – stretch and give yourself a shake before allowing the outside world to impinge on your mind.

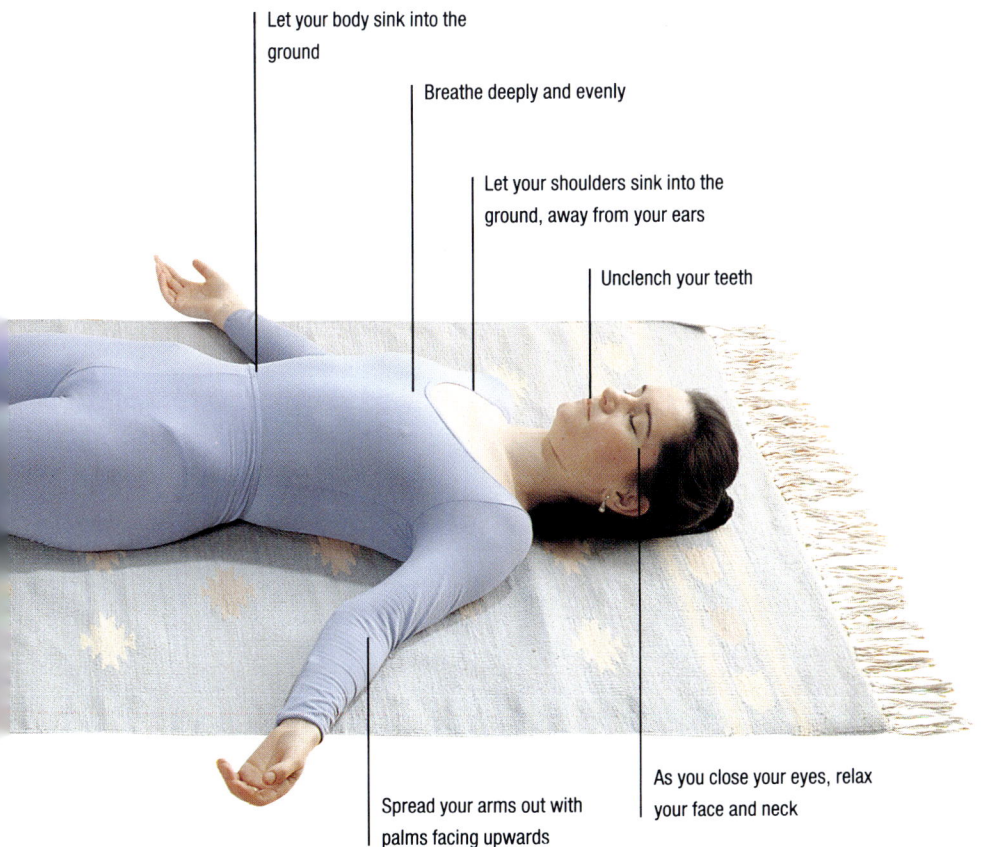

Let your body sink into the ground

Breathe deeply and evenly

Let your shoulders sink into the ground, away from your ears

Unclench your teeth

As you close your eyes, relax your face and neck

Spread your arms out with palms facing upwards

BASIC TECHNIQUES

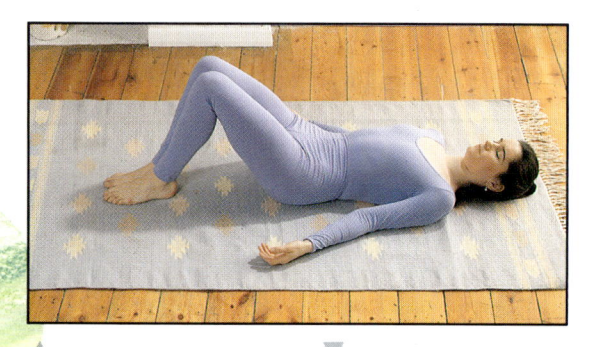

▲ If your back feels strained, try bending your legs up with your feet flat to the floor.

▼ You may find resting your legs on a chair reduces the strain on your back and makes you feel more relaxed.

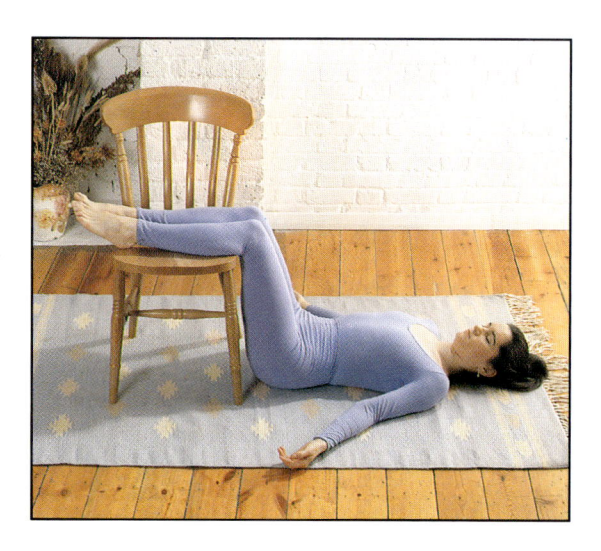

This technique can take some time to master, but you will feel the benefit from even your first attempts. To begin with, try to put aside half an hour each day to practise, or you can go through the exercises while lying in bed just before sleep. Later, as you learn precisely how to relax the various parts of the body, you will be able to let go of the tension in the muscles at will. Then you can afford to miss out the steps of tightening the muscles first. When this stage is reached any muscle that becomes tight or tense can be relaxed wherever you are – at work, driving a car or at home.

QUICK ACTION

By noticing when and where you begin to tense up, and which areas of your body are affected, you can automatically target your breathing and 'letting go' techniques for on-the-spot relief. With practice, total relaxation can be achieved in seconds, whether you are at work or in any sort of stressful situation. Shut the office door, go to the cloakroom or find a quiet corner; let yourself go completely, drain your mind of all the things you have to do, shut your eyes and concentrate on a soothing, warm, pleasant scene. If there is a crisis or row at work, switch off for a few seconds and flop, then cope.

If you find yourself becoming tense in a social situation, extricate yourself from it for a few minutes. Find a quiet corner or go to the cloakroom. Lie, sit or lean and empty your mind, concentrating on even, deep breathing as you let the tensions dissipate and disappear. Feel where the tension is and concentrate on that area, tightening the muscles, then releasing until the tension has gone. For a headache, rest your forehead on something cool and feel the point of contact draining the pain away.

Use the progressive relaxation technique if you have trouble getting to sleep. Many people have found that with practice they fall fast asleep before reaching halfway up the first leg.

ALTERNATIVE RELAXATION POSITIONS

If you need to relax but it is not possible for you to lie down, try one of the following alternatives.

Semi-reclining

Instead of lying down on something flat, half-lie in a comfortable, well-upholstered chair that has padded arms – many office chairs fit this category. Use the same relaxation technique as given above –

BASIC TECHNIQUES

close your eyes, breathe evenly and deeply, and feel the tension flowing out of your body with each breath. Allow your thoughts to drift and wander; think about how your body feels – play dead. Ten minutes of total relaxation will help you work more efficiently.

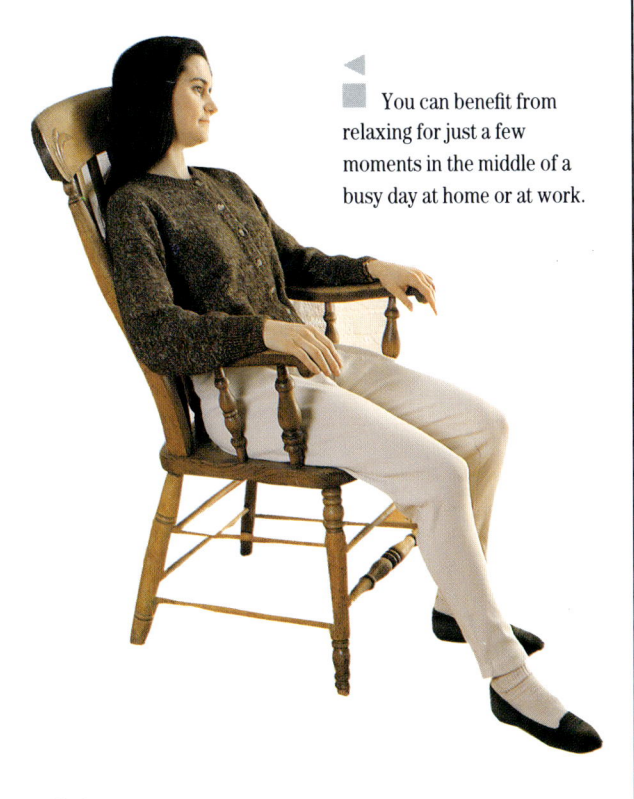

◄ You can benefit from relaxing for just a few moments in the middle of a busy day at home or at work.

Sitting
Sit on a cushion on a chair that supports your back – and, preferably, your neck. Place your hands on your lap, perhaps on another cushion placed there. Close your eyes and feel the rhythm of your breathing as your stomach moves gently in and out. Instead of tightening the muscles in your body and then relaxing them, focus on the tension in the muscles and breathe it away with each exhalation. Start with your feet and move up the body to the head. Remember to keep your head straight on the neck, as if the crown of the head is drifting towards the ceiling. When you feel completely relaxed, think of something pleasant and soothing. If you can afford the time, stay in this state for 15 minutes or so – though even five minutes will help to reduce stress.

Relaxation Checklist

Once you have mastered the basic relaxation techniques, you can apply them almost anywhere. It is important, though, to cultivate an awareness of how your body feels throughout the day, so that you can learn to recognize the difference between normal and unnatural amounts of tension. Once you begin to notice when and where you tense up, you can pinpoint your exercises to relax those muscle groups that are affected.

1 Don't leap up out of bed in the morning late, with too much to do before you start the day. Set the alarm just five minutes earlier to give yourself time to relax.

2 Plan to have time to yourself at home – when the children are at school, for example, or playing peacefully. Let the family know that certain times of the day are 'your time' – then lie down or sink into a chair and empty your mind of all household and work problems. Concentrate on how your body feels and note areas of tension; then use the relaxation technique.

3 Watch out for tension in your shoulders and arms when driving a car. Are you gripping the steering wheel, sitting bolt upright and frowning? At traffic lights or in a traffic jam, take a few seconds to concentrate on yourself: hunch the shoulders up, then let them flop down; slacken your grip on the steering wheel; relax back into your seat and feel the tension leave your body. Breathe slowly and deeply – it is difficult to become angry and frustrated while you are doing this.

BASIC TECHNIQUES

BREATHING TECHNIQUES

The importance of correct breathing has been recognised since the beginning of history. The shaman, the wise men and witch doctors of ancient times, used breathing techniques to induce trances or to improve performance, and correct breathing was, and still is, considered to be vital for good health in Eastern medicine. It is also thought to be essential if one is to progress to the higher levels of skill in meditational and martial arts and in the achievement of *asanas*, or postures taken up during t'ai chi and yoga exercises, for example. Today, it is generally recognized that correct breathing has an important role to play, in particular, in helping to reduce levels of stress, as well as its signs and symptoms.

The environmental strains of modern urban life have made breathing techniques even more important than they have been in the past, since the air that we take in to our bodies is polluted with smoke and chemicals that can damage lung tissues. Polluted air is dangerously low in oxygen – vital for the physical and mental health of the body – and low in the atmospheric ions that are linked with positive health (see 'Negative Ion Therapy', p94). Since it is impractical for the majority of us to start a new life in the less-polluted countryside, it is vitally important that we breathe as efficiently as possible.

During inspiration (breathing-in), air is drawn into the lungs, where it fills tiny air sacs that are surrounded by a network of miniscule blood vessels. The blood then absorbs the oxygen and transports it round the body to supply every cell. As the oxygen is absorbed, the blood passes carbon dioxide – the waste product of energy released from the cells – back into the air, to be removed from the body during expiration (breathing-out). If the process is less than efficient, blood oxygen levels become low, and blood carbon dioxide levels become high – too little oxygen and too much carbon dioxide and the cells will die, those of the brain and nervous system being particularly vulnerable.

The respiratory system, as the complex of muscles, nerves and tissues that performs this exchange is called, is composed of the airways – the nasal passages, pharynx, larynx, trachea (windpipe) bronchi and the lungs. The lungs have lobes: three on the right and two – to allow space for the heart – on the left. The lungs are opened up, to draw air in, by the action of the muscles beneath and around them: primarily the diaphragm, but also the intercostal muscles between the ribs. When these relax, the lungs collapse on themselves, forcing air out through the mouth and nose.

Though we all breathe by instinct, most people only use about half their lung capacity, the result being that the air sacs (alveoli) absorb too little oxygen, leaving an excess of carbon dioxide in the tissues which is reabsorbed by the blood. Conversely, panic or anxiety attacks, when breathing can become so shallow and rapid – a condition known as hyperventilation – that the body expels too much carbon dioxide, are a problem for some people. With practice, though, breathing can be made more efficient, so that hyperventilation during anxiety can be avoided by breathing control, thereby reducing stress and leading to general well-being.

Basic Method

Start by learning correct breathing techniques when lying down, alone and without distractions. Once you have mastered the technique, it can be practised in any position, anywhere – eventually it will become a habit.

1. Put on loose, comfortable clothes and lie on your back on the floor, using a mat if more comfortable, or on your bed.

2. Place both your hands on the lower edges of your ribs, with the fingers nearly touching.

BASIC TECHNIQUES

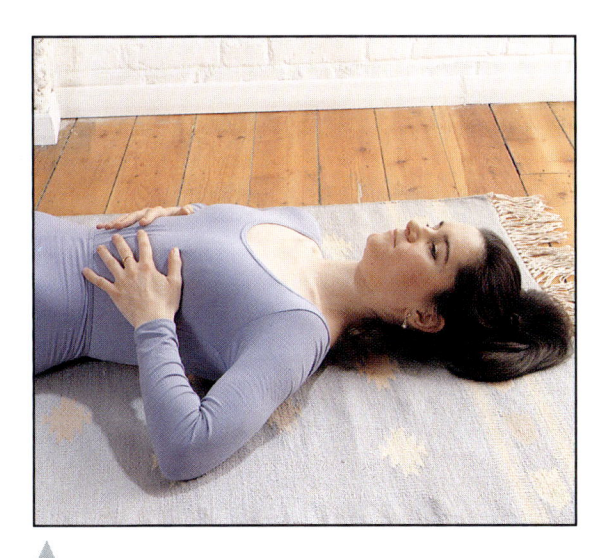

▲ As you inhale, your fingers will move up and apart.

3 Relax your body (*see* 'Basic Relaxation Technique', *p56*).

4 Breathe in deeply and smoothly through your nostrils. Feel your diaphragm pulling out and down, your stomach rising and your ribs expanding upwards and outwards. Hold the breath for a few seconds.

5 Breathe out smoothly. This requires no muscular activity, since all that happens is that the diaphragm and muscles of the chest let go, but try to ensure that all the air that you inhaled is expelled. The ribs collapse down and in; the stomach lowers.

6 Repeat three or four times, then relax and breathe naturally for a few minutes, before starting the sequence again.

WATCHPOINT

If you feel heady or faint during the breathing exercises, relax and breathe naturally for a few minutes – the sensation passes quickly, and is the result of the brain receiving an unusually large amount of oxygen.

WATCHPOINT

Your shoulders should remain stationary during breathing. Many people, especially women, breathe solely into their upper lobes by raising and lowering their shoulders. This does not give the body an adequate supply of oxygen, and is a common symptom of stress.

Alternative Methods

Since correct breathing can make a significant difference to how you feel, it is worth practising in different positions and situations.

Sitting

1 Make sure you are sitting comfortably, with your spine straight.

2 Relax your shoulders and place your hands loosely on your lap.

3 Breathe using the same basic method as for lying down.

4 Feel the air filling your lungs, right down to the bottom lobes.

5 Check your shoulders – they should not be moving up and down.

6 If you feel that you are not filling your lungs fully, place your hands on the bottom edge of the ribs and over the stomach and check that your ribs and stomach are expanding fully under your fingers as you breathe in. Breathe like this a few times until you sense the movement and then return your hands to your lap.

Walking

1 Walk at a steady pace, letting your hands swing loosely by your side.

2 Breathe in deeply – as in the basic method – for a certain number of paces, hold the breath for half that number and breathe out gradually for the same number. Find which number of paces feels right for you.

3 Maintain the rhythm and repeat the exercise five times. Then relax and breathe naturally.

4 Repeat the whole exercise a few times during each walk.

THE ABDOMINAL PUSH

This is a forced expiration caused by a firm contraction of the abdominal muscles. Strictly speaking, it is not a breathing exercise, but it does help to build up awareness of the movement of the abdomen and diaphragm during respiration. It also helps to rid the lower air sacs of carbon dioxide and is useful as a pick-me-up if you have been sitting stationary for a long time – perhaps after a journey.

1 Lie down as for the basic method, though once the technique is learnt it can be performed sitting or standing.

2 Completely relax the whole body.

3 Inhale through the nostrils quickly and deeply, so that the stomach swells. Place your hands on the stomach if it helps to feel the movement.

4 Straightaway pull the stomach muscles in hard and down – as though trying to squash them against the spine – forcing the air out through your nostrils. If necessary, jerk them in and down again. Each breath should take no more than three seconds.

5 Do not use your chest or shoulders, only the stomach muscles.

6 Concentrate on the up and down movement of the abdomen.

7 Repeat eight times and then breathe naturally for a minute or two before starting again.

A TENSION RELAXER

This exercise is particularly useful, since it only takes a few minutes and can be performed anywhere.

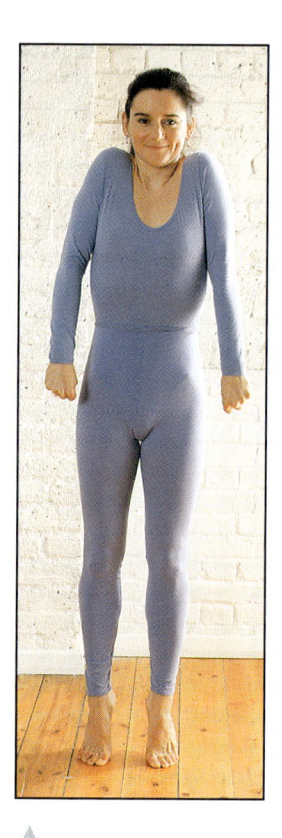

1 Stand up with your hands hanging loosely by your side.

2 Breathe in slowly through your nostrils, tensing all your muscles at the same time.

3 Hunch your shoulders up to your ears, clench your hands as hard as possible, tighten your stomach muscles, clench your buttocks and raise yourself up on to tiptoe.

4 Hold this position to the count of five. Fix your eye on something straight ahead to help your balance.

5 Slowly breathe out through your nostrils and at the same time relax all your muscles, so that by the time you have fully exhaled your shoulders are down, your hands are floppy, your stomach is relaxed and your knees are slightly bent.

6 Repeat five times.

▲ Clench your muscles and stand on tiptoe as in stage 3 of the Tension Relaxer.

The Healing Breath

This method of healing is used in all branches of Eastern medicine, though not in orthodox Western medicine. It involves breathing in the *chi*, as Chinese and Japanese medicine calls the 'life force', or the *prana*, as Indian medicine names it, into the lungs and visualizing it flowing from them first into the solar plexus and then to the area to be healed. During exhalation the disease is visualized flowing out of the body. If you wish to try this, use either the basic technique or the sun and moon technique.

Sun and Moon Breath

This breathing technique is recommended for calming the spirit and the mind. The sun and moon are seen here as symbols of the positive and negative, and this technique shows you how to inhale the positive energy of the sun and exhale the negative waste products of the body. You can do this to calm and refresh yourself in the office or while travelling.

1 Sit in an upright position – cross-legged if you can manage it, otherwise sit on a firm-backed chair.

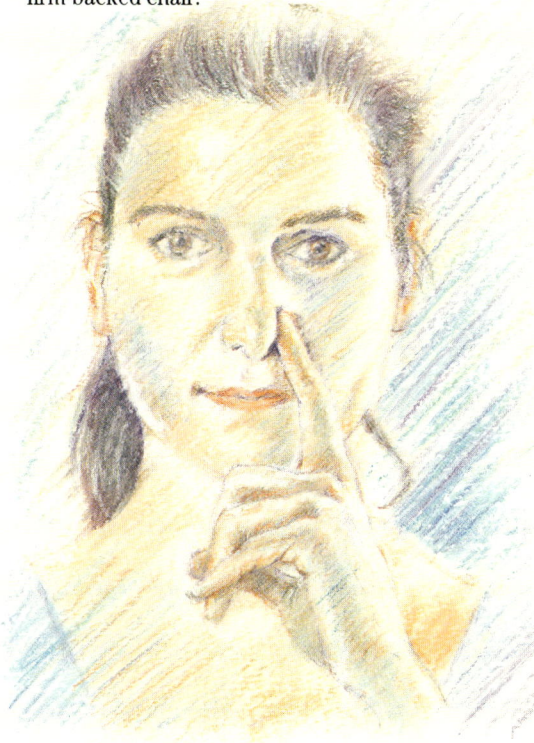

2 Pinch your nostrils shut with your right hand, the thumb closing the right nostril and the index and middle finger closing the left nostril. Only gentle pressure is needed, so do not pinch too hard.

3 Breathe through your mouth as you practise opening and closing the nostrils alternately.

4 When you have learnt how to do this, inhale deeply and slowly as for the basic method through your right nostril – keep the left nostril firmly closed.

5 Hold for the amount of time it took you to inhale – though not if it feels uncomfortable.

6 Exhale gradually through your left nostril, again for the same length of time it took to inhale. The comparative ratio for these three motions – breathing in, holding, then breathing out – is therefore 1:1:1. This rhythm can take a while to master, but the control it engenders and the results are worthwhile. Traditionally, those advanced in yoga use a ratio of 1:4:2, but without specialized training you should not try to go beyond 1:2:2.

7 Breathe in this way five times and then use the left nostril to inhale and the right nostril to exhale and repeat.

8 Breathe twice through both nostrils deeply and fully.

9 Relax totally in the same position and feel the tension disappearing.

BASIC TECHNIQUES

POSTURE

Correct posture is vital for mental and physical well-being. Many people, often as a reflection of their attitudes to life or as a response to stress, hold their bodies incorrectly. This is doubly unfortunate: first, bad posture can cause others to relate negatively; second, bad posture can increase the stress that it may be reflecting by contributing to excess muscular tension. In any event, it is difficult to feel confident and out-going if you are slouched or hunched over.

However, with a little practice and application you can correct your posture, relieve stress, feel confident and give others a positive impression of your personality. Correct posture means standing erect and stable, with the feet nearly together, the arms hanging relaxed by your side and the pelvis, spine, neck and head straight, but not rigid; the crown of the head should be the uppermost point of the body. The two most common errors of posture are slouching and standing over-erect. The slouched position – often with rounded shoulders, a caved-in chest and protruding stomach – prevents deep breathing, attracts back trouble and leads to a pessimistic outlook on life. The over-erect, or 'military' bearing – with exaggerated spinal curves, a pigeon chest and your nose in the air – crushes the spine, causing back and neck problems, and is often the stance adopted by an over-controlled personality, who inwardly lacks confidence.

If you are particularly interested in techniques which will help you hold yourself well and move well see Alexander Technique (p102), Feldenkrais Method (p108) and Yoga (p110).

Method
Stand up straight and check your posture from the front and side with mirrors – or ask a friend to look for you. Compare your posture with that shown in the illustrations on these pages.

For a correct posture:

1 the crown of your head should be high – pull your hair straight up at the crown and feel how the head lifts towards the ceiling.

2 your chin should be level, not sticking up or tucked in.

3 your neck should be straight, with no lump sticking out at the nape of the neck.

4 your chest should be broad and open, not collapsed or thrust out.

5 your spine should be straight, with gentle not exaggerated curves.

6 your hips should be square to your shoulders, the bottom neither thrust out nor tucked in exaggeratedly.

7 your legs should be firm, with the weight of the body evenly distributed to each foot.

8 your feet should be in line with your legs, with your weight carried on the whole length of the foot, from the heel down the outside curve to the base of all the toes – like a two-sided triangle.

The overall effect should be one of poise and freedom. This posture is the basis for all body positions and movements: lying, sitting, walking, running. The basic posture will help, too, when you are lifting, pushing or carrying, by preventing injury. Always remember that the legs are the powerhouse of the body and that all lifting, pushing and pulling should be performed by use of the leg muscles, and not by straining the spine.

Following these steps, thinking about how you are holding your body, can in itself be a relaxation technique as it focusses your attention inward. Try working through these steps while standing in a queue or waiting for a train. You can calm yourself and improve your posture at the same time.

BASIC TECHNIQUES

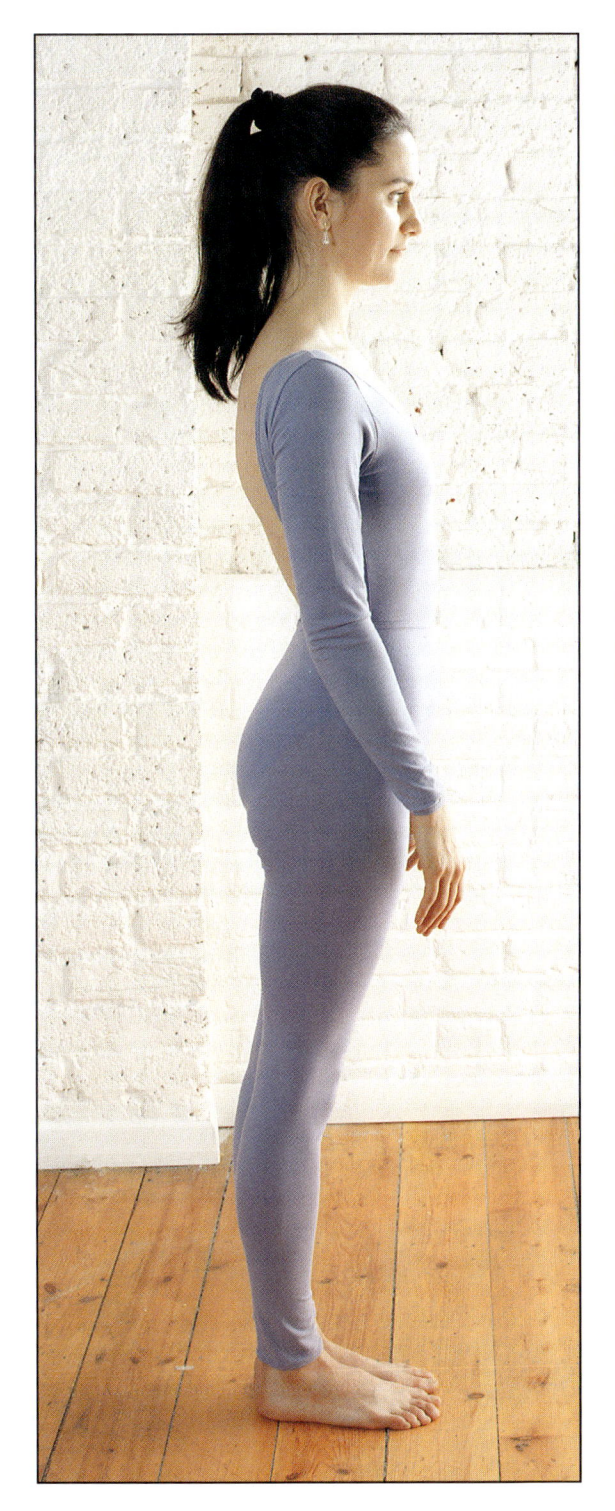

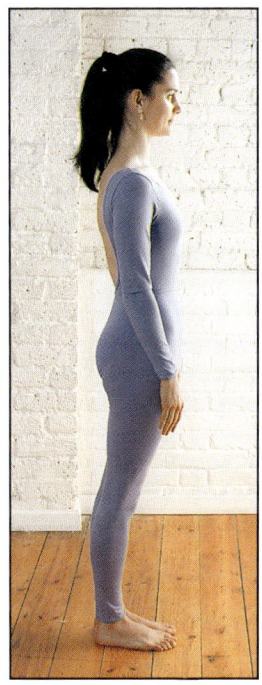

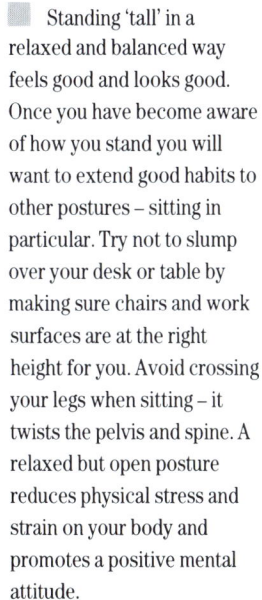

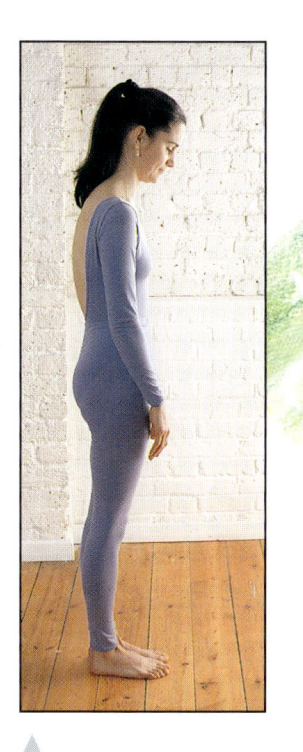

▲ Standing 'tall' in a relaxed and balanced way feels good and looks good. Once you have become aware of how you stand you will want to extend good habits to other postures – sitting in particular. Try not to slump over your desk or table by making sure chairs and work surfaces are at the right height for you. Avoid crossing your legs when sitting – it twists the pelvis and spine. A relaxed but open posture reduces physical stress and strain on your body and promotes a positive mental attitude.

▲ Slouching with a caved-in chest and rounded shoulders presents an unattractive and depressing picture, and prevents deep breathing.

◀ Standing 'over-erect' is thought by some people to be a desirable posture but in fact it causes an exaggerated curve in the spine, and back and neck problems.

BASIC TECHNIQUES

WARMING-UP AND STRETCHING EXERCISES

It is a good principle to warm up and stretch before beginning any form of strenuous exercise and the sequences below can be used for this. However they are also beneficial in their own right. Gentle exercise – and stretching in particular – is one of the easiest and most effective ways of quietening an over-active mind, refreshing a tired body and generally aiding relaxation. The exercises on these pages can be done at any time.

▶ Begin by standing straight with your feet parallel and about shoulder-width apart, hands hanging loosely at your side. If possible stand by an open window and take a few deep breaths to fill and empty the lungs. Bend forward as far as you can. Relax into the pose then raise your body bringing the head up first. Take some more deep breaths.

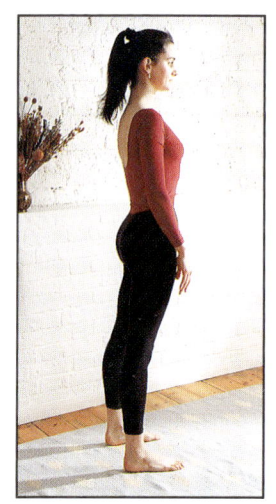

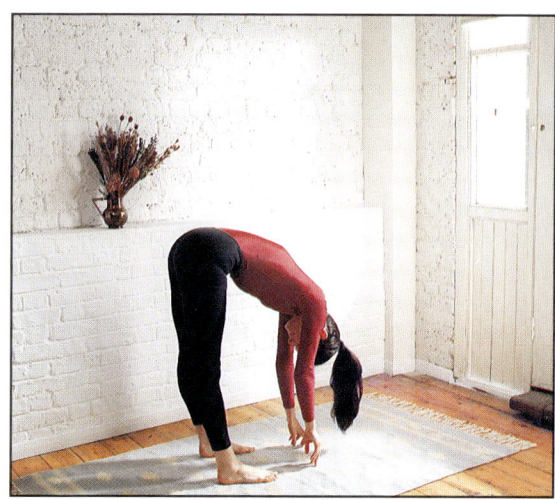

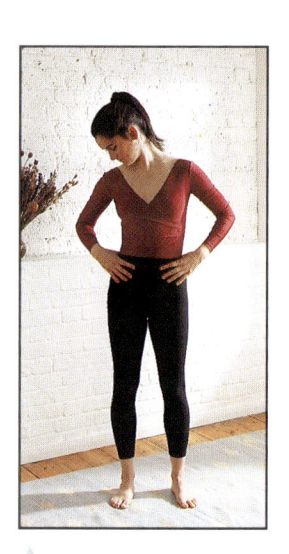

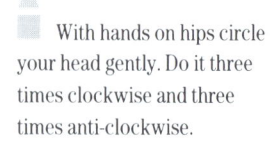

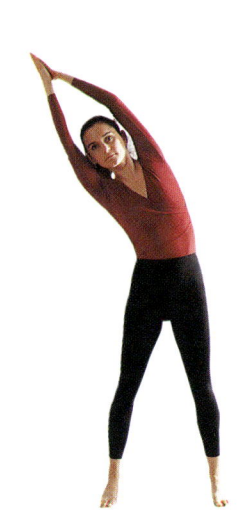

▲ With hands on hips circle your head gently. Do it three times clockwise and three times anti-clockwise.

▲ Stand with feet slightly wider apart. Put your hands above your head palms together. Bend gently to the right and relax into the pose. Return to the upright then repeat to the left. Do this four times.

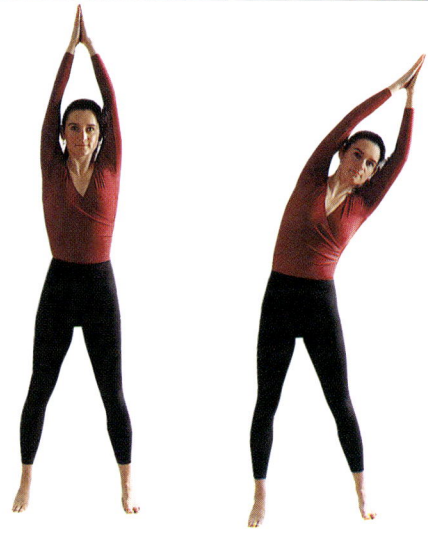

66

BASIC TECHNIQUES

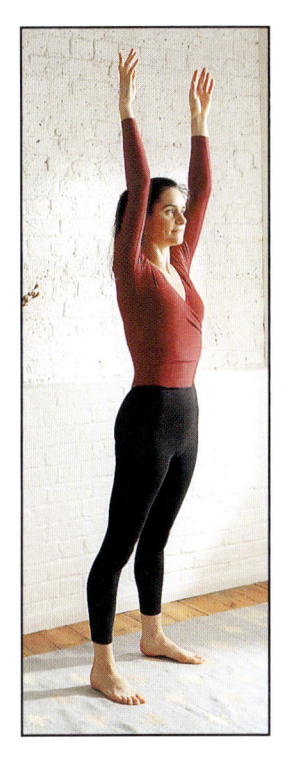

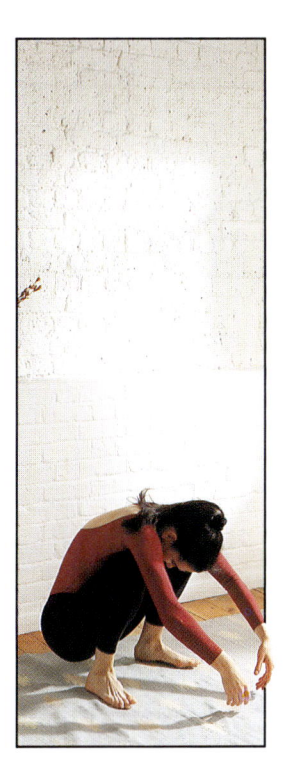

▶ Stand with feet parallel and shoulder-width apart. Stretch your arms above your head making sure you feel the stretch right through your body. Move slowly down into a crouch then gradually stretch up again. Repeat three times.

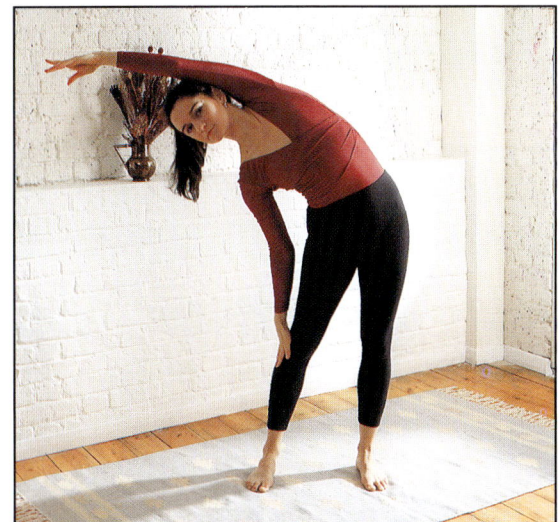

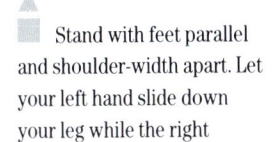

▲ Stand with feet parallel and shoulder-width apart. Let your left hand slide down your leg while the right stretches over the head pulling your shoulders to the left. Keep your legs and hips still. Repeat three times.

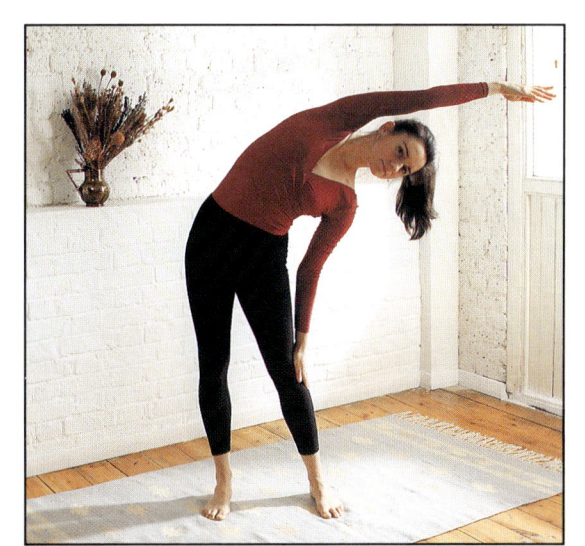

▲ Do the same movement with the right hand moving down and the left stretching over the head. Really feel and enjoy the stretch through the left side. Again repeat three times.

BASIC TECHNIQUES

Morning Stretches

Try to set aside ten minutes each morning to stretch and warm up your muscles for the day ahead. Breathe deeply as you exercise. You can begin by stretching your arms and legs even before you get out of bed.

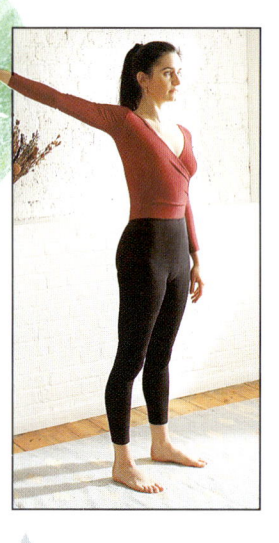

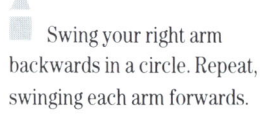

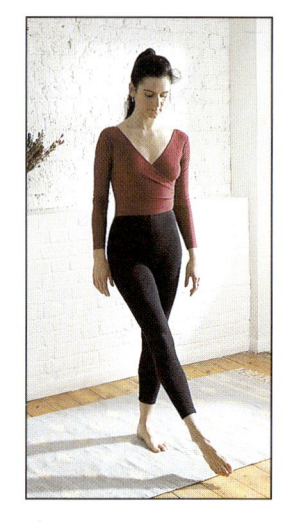

▲ Swing your right arm backwards in a circle. Repeat, swinging each arm forwards.

▲ Standing as for the previous exercises swing each leg, in turn, backwards and forwards.

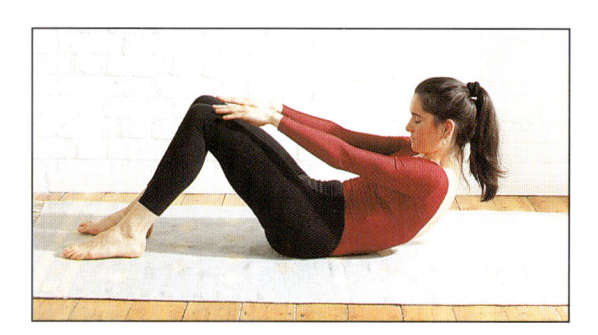

▲ Lie on the floor with your legs bent, feet flat on the floor. Slowly raise your head and shoulders until your hands touch your knees. Lower yourself gently and repeat five times.

During the day

▷ Don't forget to stand up and stretch during the day at work, at home or on a long plane or train journey. It will help relieve tension and keep you feeling relaxed and alert. Stand with feet parallel and shoulder-width apart. Interlock your fingers in front of you and raise your arms turning the palms upwards. Feel the stretch equally down both sides of the body.

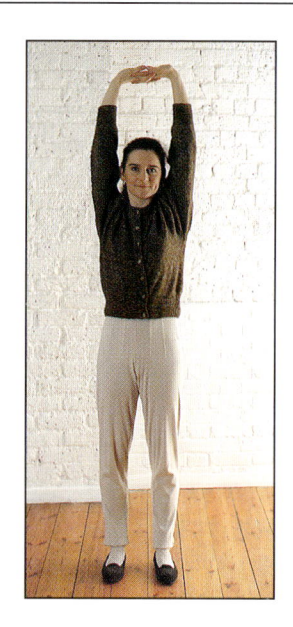

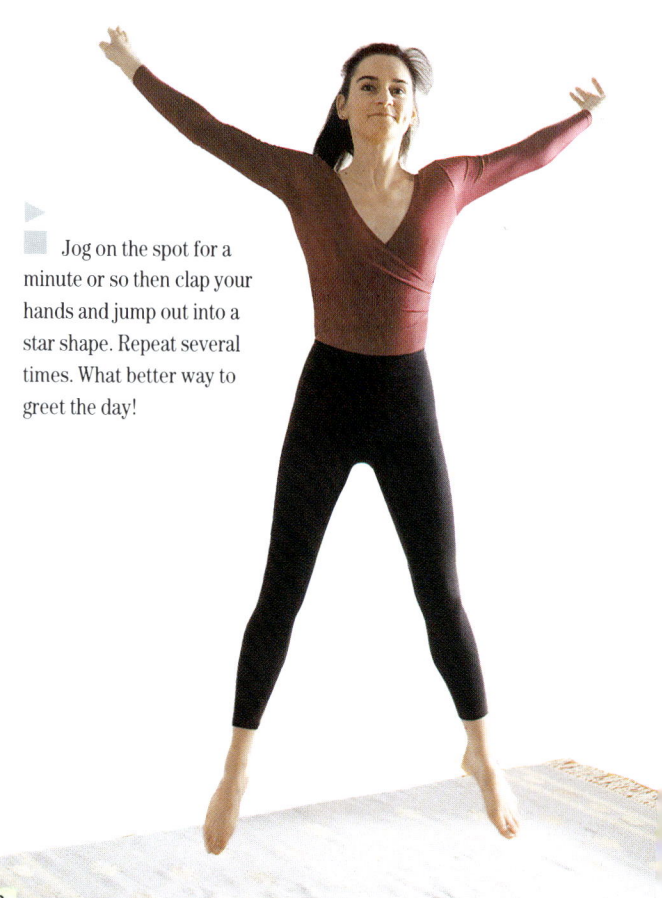

▷ Jog on the spot for a minute or so then clap your hands and jump out into a star shape. Repeat several times. What better way to greet the day!

BASIC TECHNIQUES

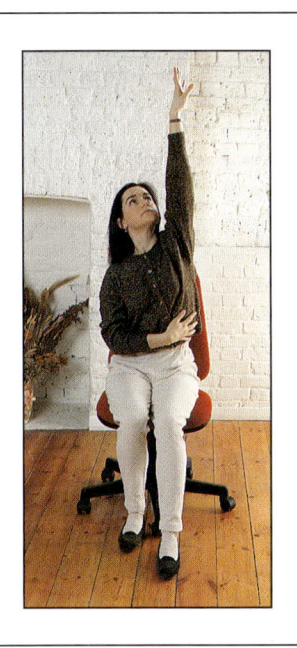

▲ You can even do a few stretching exercises when you are completely chair-bound. Stretch up your left arm as high as you can. Stretch the whole left side right up to the fingertips. Repeat for the right side. If there's room stretch each leg, in turn, out in front of you. Concentrate on stretching right to the tip of the big toe. Repeat as often as you like.

Evening Stretches
To unwind at the end of the day stretching is an ideal form of exercise. It will calm an over-active mind and make you feel pleasantly tired rather than exhausted and irritable.

▼ Lie on the floor with legs bent and feet flat to the ground. Roll gently from side to side. Let your left hand come over to the right side of the knees. Repeat several times on both sides.

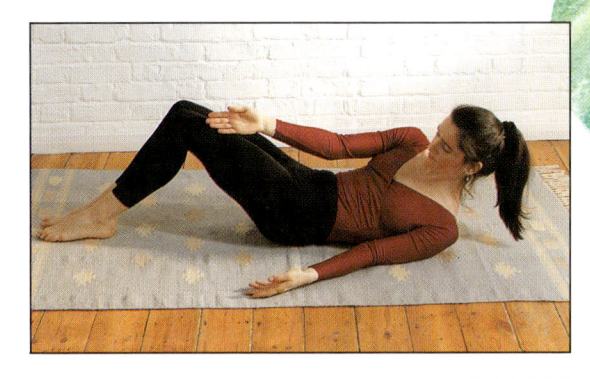

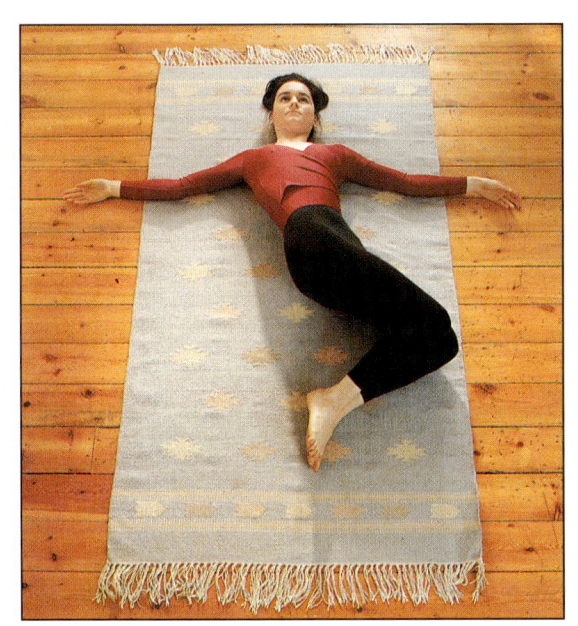

▲ Lie on the floor with legs bent and feet flat to the ground. Spread your arms wide. Let your legs fall over to the right. Feel the stretch then centre them and let them fall to the left. Repeat several times.

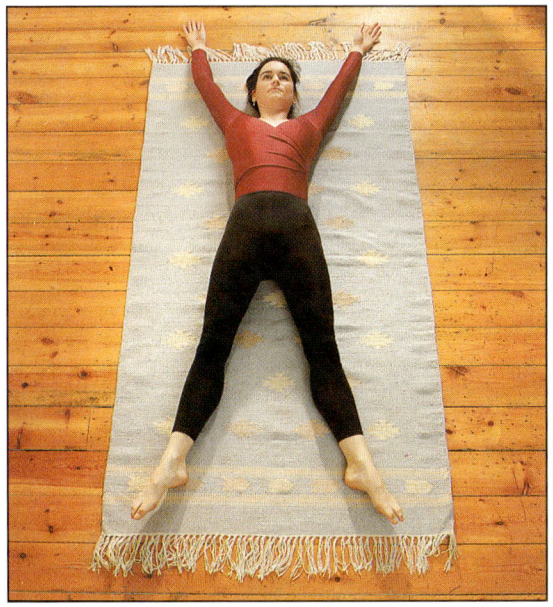

▲ Lie on your back and stretch your hands above your head. Feel the stretch right through your body from finger tips to toes. End with the basic relaxation technique (p56).

RELAXATION TECHNIQUES

To many people, relaxation does not come naturally – though stress does. Because of this, most people have to make a special effort to learn how to relax.

Choose from any combination of the techniques described, until you find those that suit you and your lifestyle; when you try any particular one, concentrate on what you personally want out of it, and remember that you are more likely to succeed if you choose a method that has a special appeal to you.

Some of the techniques described have primarily a mental effect; others mainly affect the body. Many of the mental techniques originate in the East, where they have been used for centuries to achieve deep relaxation, inner peace and tranquillity. If you feel that such qualities are missing in your life try one of these techniques – meditation, for example.

Other techniques are based on achieving a physical harmony and balance that will, in turn, affect mental well-being: if you find it easier to achieve physical and mental relaxation through movement or 'doing something', these are the techniques for you.

Whichever techniques you choose, persevere with them for a while before trying another technique – quick changes are in themselves a sign of stress. But do read through the other techniques: they contain many useful hints which may help in your overall programme.

TECHNIQUES

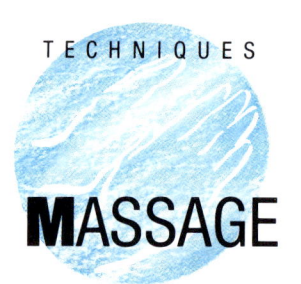

MASSAGE

The therapeutic use of the sense of touch, either by oneself or by another. Touching is not just therapeutic, though, but necessary for a normal, happy life. By instinct we all touch or rub a painful area to give relief, and we hug to give comfort and affection. Unfortunately, as we grow out of childhood we tend to formalize touch, confusing it with sexuality, and lose the benefits to be gained from contact with other people. Children who have been deprived of physical contact during their early years often develop severe psychological problems in later life, while adults become withdrawn and introverted without touch, finding it difficult to let go and relax for fear of appearing childish.

Massage is a fairly recent name for the old-established art of healing by touch – ancient Chinese, Indian and Egyptian writers all describe it as a method of maintaining health and curing disease. Different names have been used in different cultures, though: the Greek physician Hippocrates talked of *anatripsis*, while others have referred to "rubbing", "manipulation" and even "shampooing". Massage is also an important part of the Indian technique of Ayurdevic treatment, where all members of a family are taught to massage each other.

Therapeutic massage as we know it today was first developed by a Swede called Per Henrik Ling (1776–1839). His ideas spread quickly throughout Europe and

MEDICAL ALERT

Massage should not be attempted in cases of inflammation, fever, contagious disease, heart conditions, or in cases of thrombosis or phlebitis where there is the risk of disturbing an existing blood clot.

TECHNIQUES

Effleurage
Stroking with the whole hand, keeping the fingers relaxed. The basic stroke of massage, this is used to relax the superficial muscles at the start of a massage and to relax and soothe at the end; it is also used as a connecting movement, when, having finished working on one part of the body, the masseuse moves on to another. Sometimes vigorous effleurage is given to stimulate the skin and the circulation.

Pettrisage
Kneading, squeezing and rolling the fleshy areas of the body in a rhythmical, rocking movement. The technique is similar to that used to knead dough, though it can be either deep and firm or superficial. Pettrisage is effective on the shoulders, hips, buttocks and legs, toning and stretching the muscles to relieve stiffness and tension. It also improves the circulation and assists the dispersal of toxins from the tissues.

Effleurage

Pettrisage

there are still Swedish Institutes in many cities – that is why therapeutic massage is still sometimes called 'Swedish massage'. At the end of the last century, it was common for medical practitioners to prescribe a course of massage; the people who performed such therapeutic massages eventually formed a society of masseuses and masseurs – the precursor of The Chartered Society of Physiotherapists – to regulate the profession and distinguish its services from those offered by less-well-intentioned ladies. Unfortunately, as medicine became more scientific during the 20th century, the use of massage, though still taught to all physiotherapists, became too time-consuming to be frequently prescribed. However, today massage is making a comeback in the approach to terminal care and psychological problems.

Massage is applied directly to the muscles and ligaments of the body, but has a secondary effect on the circulatory and nervous systems. It relieves muscle tension, breaks down adhesions between tissues and improves circulation and lymph drainage – thus helping the body to rid itself of toxins. Massage can relieve pain by stimulating the production of hormones called endorphins – the body's own painkillers – and, by increasing the sensory input to the brain, blocking out the transmission of the pain messages. Its effect on the nervous system is to calm, soothe and give an overall sense of well-being, making it a wonderful method of combating the symptoms of stress that our hectic lifestyles produce. This is an ideal relaxation technique for busy people as you don't need a regular class.

Friction
Deep circulatory movements, using the thumbs, to break down adhesions between tissues or specific knots of tension. Friction can be painful – if it is too painful, the masseuse should stop. The area to be treated is usually relaxed with pettrisage first, then massaged using friction every so often, in order that the knot is broken down gradually rather than in one go. Friction should never be used on the spine itself, but only on the muscles running down either side of the spine.

Tapotement
A percussive movement on the skin. Percussion consists of cupping, pummelling, hacking, flicking and clapping the fleshy parts of the body to stimulate, invigorate and warm. (Tapotement should not be used on bony areas of the body, such as the spine and shins.) This improves the circulation and reduces tension in the muscles. If used as part of a relaxation massage, it should be followed by effleurage.

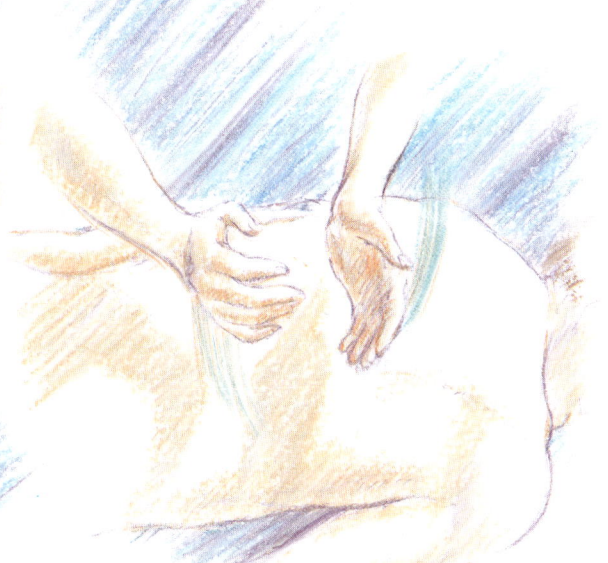

Tapotement

Friction

TECHNIQUES

Facial massage

Stress and tension often have their first visible signs in rigidity of the facial muscles, with tightness in the brow, jaw and eyes. A relaxing face massage can help to remove this tension, bringing a glow to the complexion and a general sense of well-being. The recipient of the massage should be lying down with their head flat. The giver kneels behind the head. Before starting the massage, the giver should apply a few drops of oil to the fingers (normally a vegetable-based kind mixed with a couple of drops of almond oil) to coat them lightly with a thin film of oil.

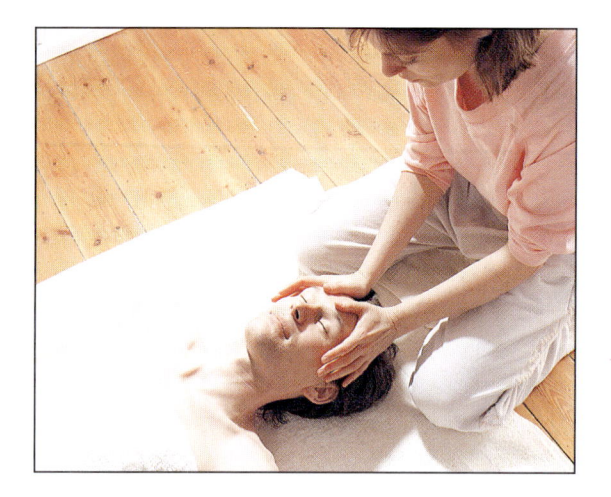

◁ 1 Start at the forehead, with the thumbs in the upper centre, and the fingers at the side of the head. Press firmly and evenly, stroking the thumbs gently outwards from the centre of the brow area to the temples.

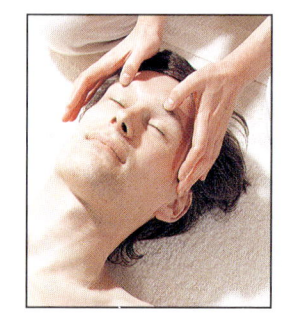

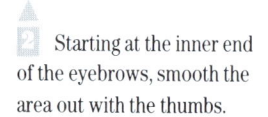

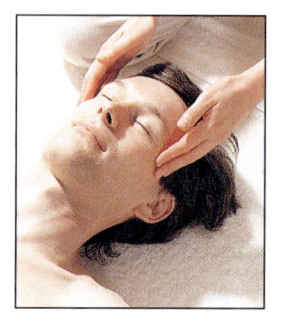

▲ 2 Starting at the inner end of the eyebrows, smooth the area out with the thumbs.

▲ 3 Massage the temple area with small circular motions of the fingers.

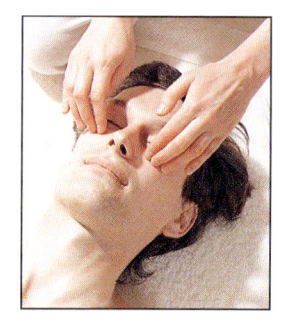

▲ 4 Using the tips of the fingers, press gently around the fleshy area under the eye.

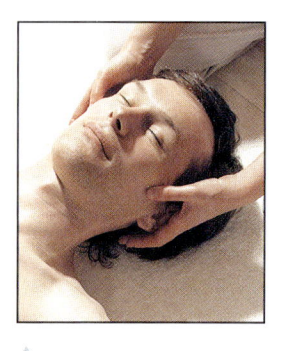

▲ 5 Then stroke the cheeks with the thumbs moving from the nose area across the cheekbone towards the ears.

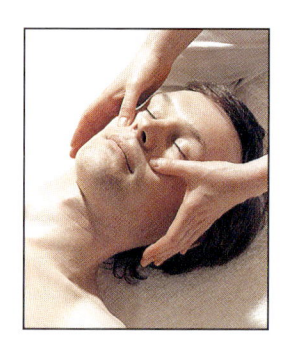

▲ 6 Press with the thumbs under the cheekbones from the nose towards the ears.

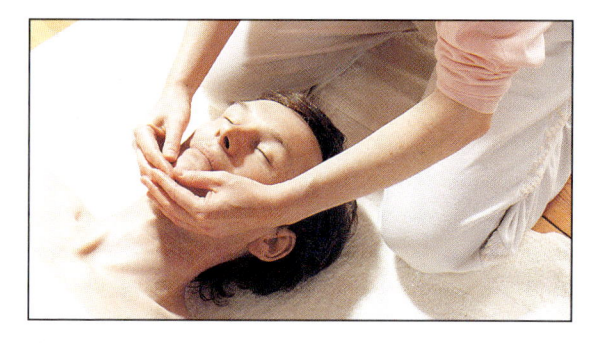

▲ 7 At the jawline, cup the hands under the chin, drawing the hands out along the lower jaw in a stroking motion up to the point where the jaw bone meets the lobe of the ear

74

MASSAGE

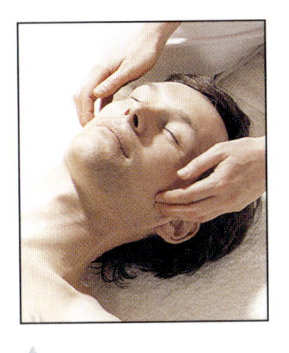

▲ 8 Using the fingertips, massage the jaw angle with small circular motions.

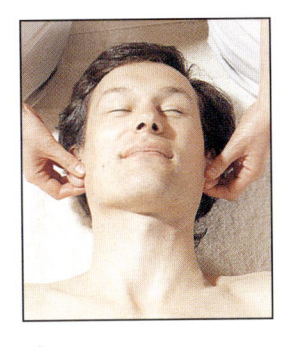

▲ 9 Gently squeeze the ears around the outer edge from the ear lobe to the top and back, using fingertips.

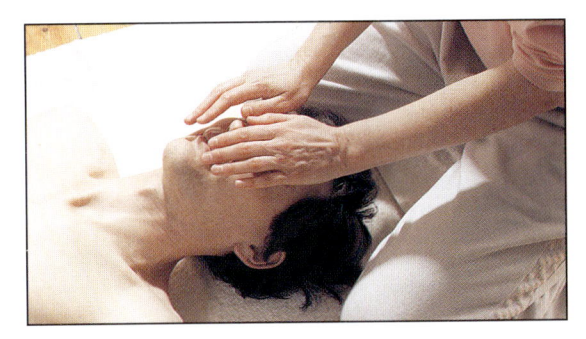

▲ 10 To end the massage gently, rest the palms of the hands over the recipient's eyes for a few seconds.

Quick Massage

This can be done anywhere – in a straight-backed chair in the office, for example – and is particularly useful for relieving tension in the neck and shoulder areas. It also helps to relieve stress-related headaches.

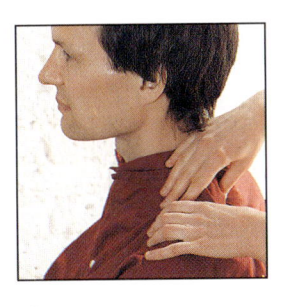

▲ 1 Knead with the thumbs in a circular motion along the shoulder line to the neck.

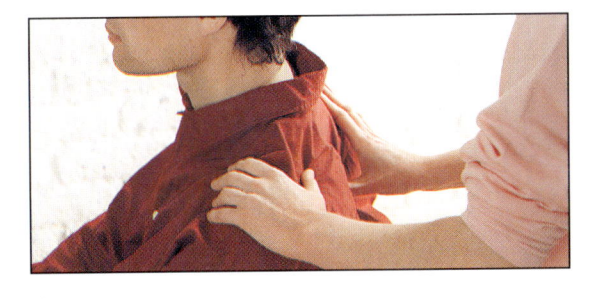

▲ 2 Still using the thumbs, press down along the muscle alongside the upper part of the spinal column. Repeat steps 1 and 2 on the other side of the body.

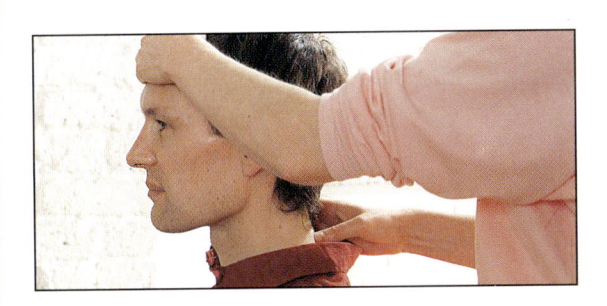

▲ 3 Returning to the other side of the body, press down with the thumbs at the base of the neck moving up towards the base of the skull.

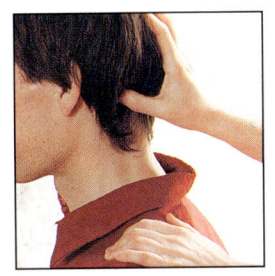

▲ 4 Press with the thumbs along the base of the skull upwards.

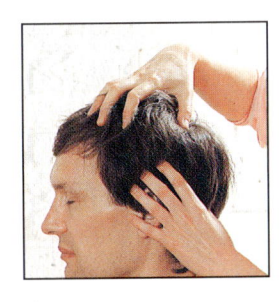

▲ 5 Finish by using a "shampooing" motion over the whole head.

TECHNIQUES

Back massage
The back is usually the starting point for a whole body massage. To conduct the massage, sit with the knees either side of the recipient's head. Oil the hands with a little massage oil.

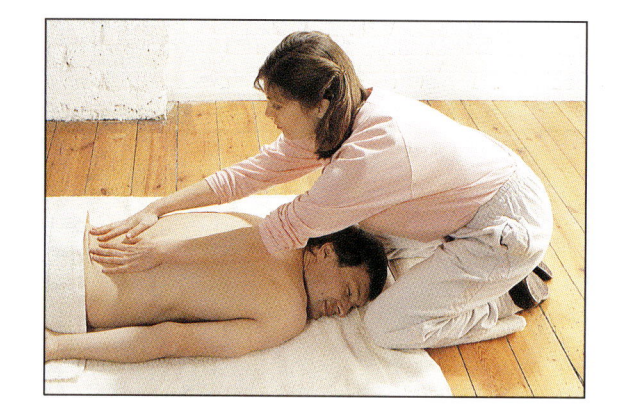

▶ 1 Start with long even strokes of the whole hand down the length of the back, from the upper back to the base of the spine. This helps to spread the oil and relaxes the recipient for the rest of the massage.

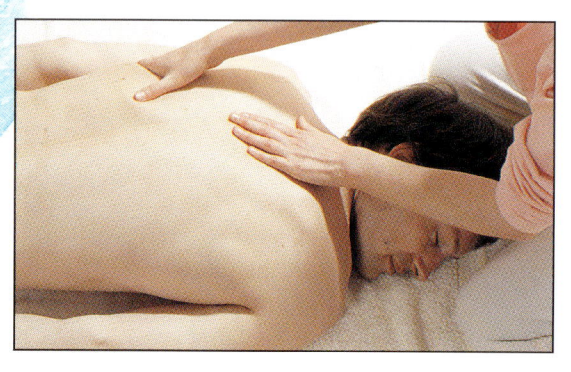

▲ 2 Move across to one shoulder area (the opposite side to the way the head is lying) and rhythmically squeeze and knead the flesh around the blade area.

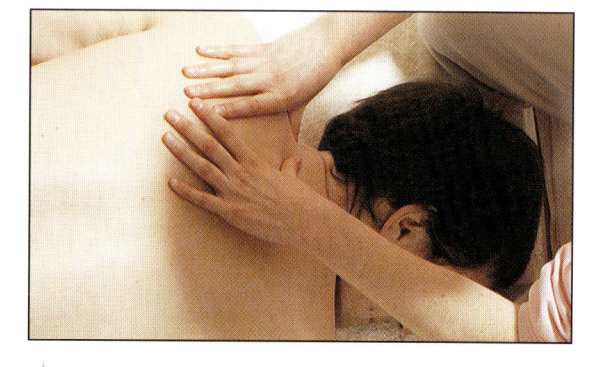

▲ 3 Using the thumbs, and small, firm strokes, work the triangle between the shoulder blade and spine. Then roll the thumbs down the muscle alongside the spine. Repeat 1–3 on the other side.

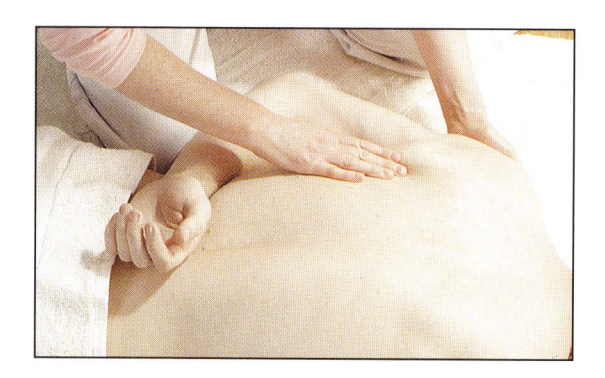

▲ 4 Moving to the lower back, squeeze and knead from the top of the buttocks to the shoulder area. Rest the hands on the lower back to finish.

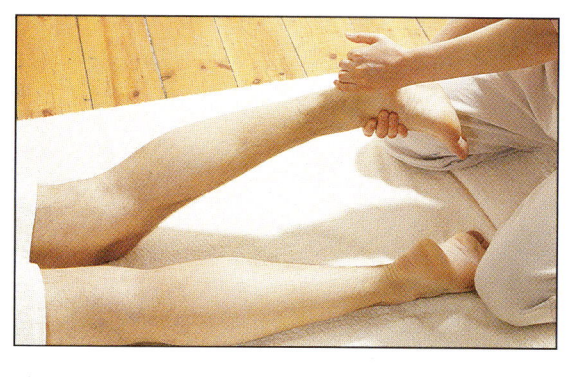

▲ 5 With one hand cupping the heel, the other around the top of the foot, gently pull the leg to stretch the joints of the leg and lower back. Repeat on the other side.

MASSAGE

Front Massage

The recipient turns on to their back. Oil your hands again, and sit as for the start of the back massage.

▶

1 Starting with the neck area, stroke the hands alternately along the back of the neck to turn the recipient's head gently from side to side.

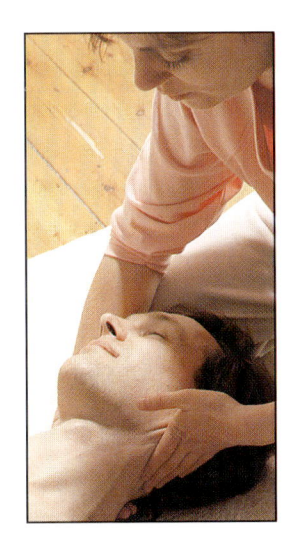

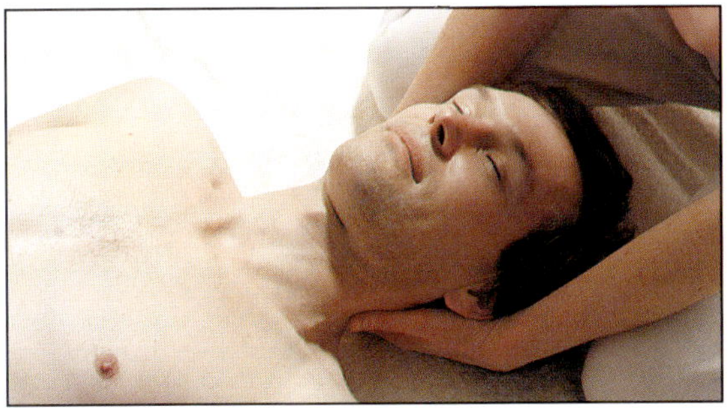

▲

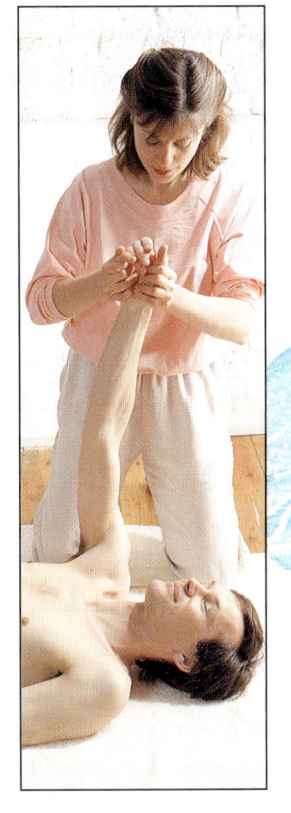

2 Stretch the neck a little by cupping both hands under the base of the skull, gently pulling the recipient's head.

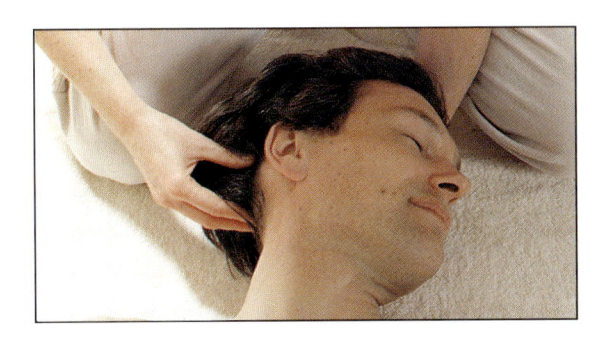

▲

3 Cupping the head gently turn the neck to one side and press along the base of the skull from the centre towards the ear. Then use a "shampooing" motion.

▶

4 Taking the recipient's hand, gently lift the arm and stretch it up at right angles to the body. Repeat on the other side.

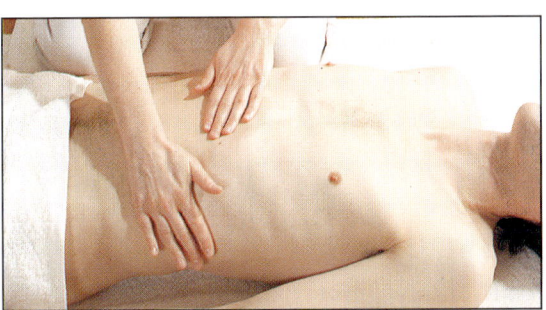

▲

5 With the palms of the hands circle the stomach and lower abdomen with clockwise motions. Finish the massage by gently holding the recipient's feet.

TECHNIQUES

Self massage

Although self message is by no means as relaxing as being given a massage it is still an excellent way to treat tension, and can be done while sitting in a chair, if necessary, or during a break in a long journey. Massaging the neck and shoulder region can often relieve tension headaches more effectively than painkillers. Take off your shoes and loosen any tight clothing.

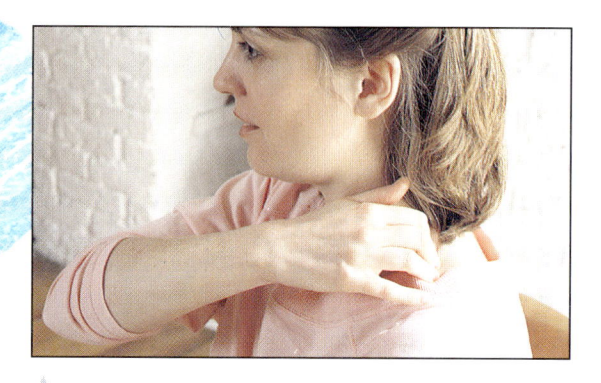

▲ 1 Press down with the finger tips in small circling movements on the muscle running from the shoulder to the base of the neck. Do both sides.

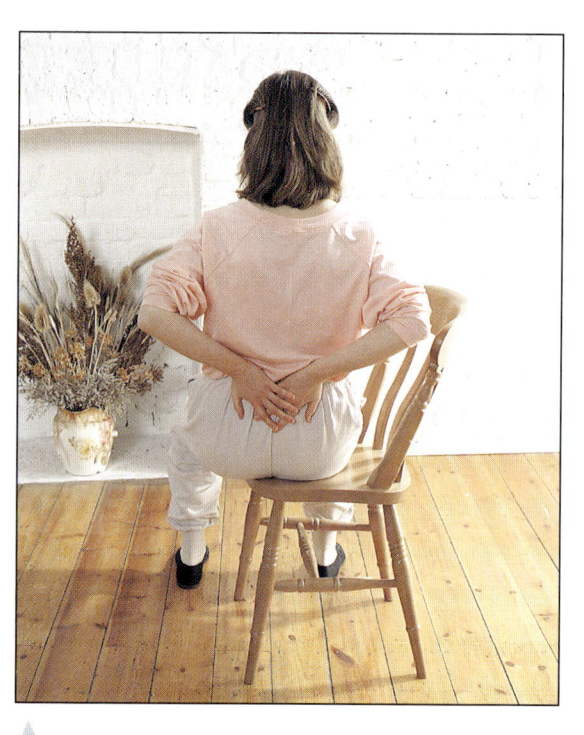

▲ 2 Sitting sideways in a chair, press both hands together on the lower back, and circle them in an anti-clockwise direction.

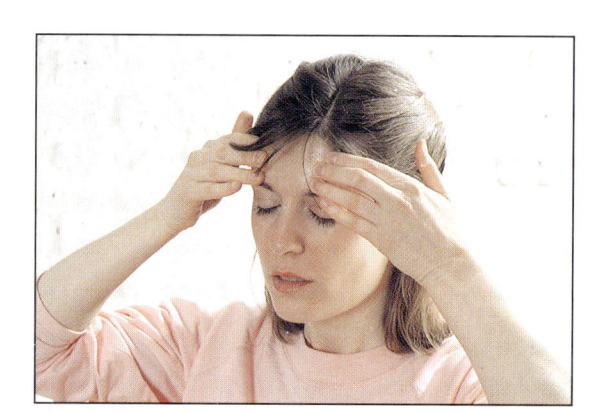

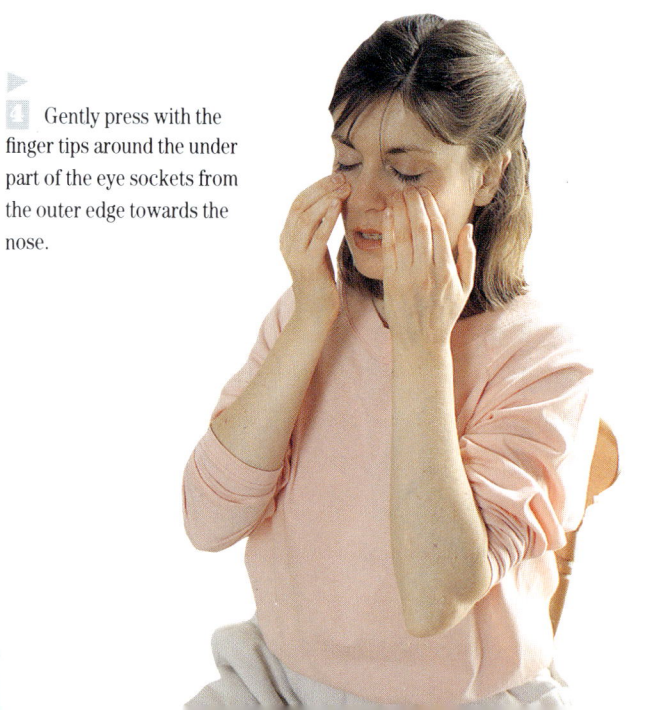

▲ 3 Press gently around the brow area, starting with the centre of the forehead, drawing the fingertips out towards the hairline.

▶ 4 Gently press with the finger tips around the under part of the eye sockets from the outer edge towards the nose.

MASSAGE

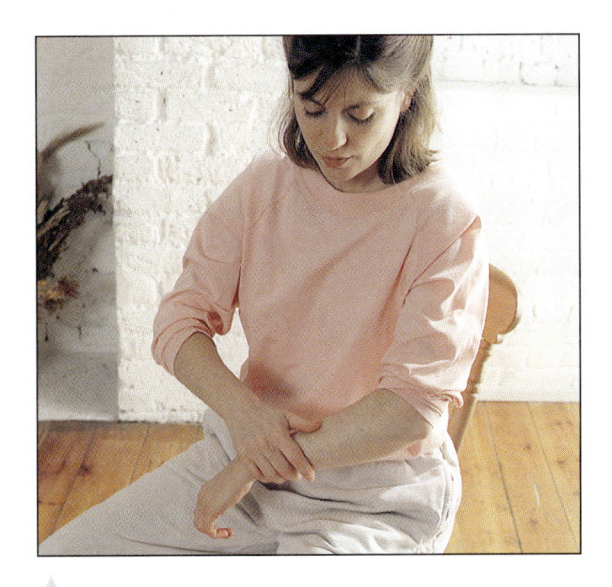

5 Using the whole hand, starting at the top of the upper arm, scrunch the muscles all the way down the arm to the wrist and off through the hand.

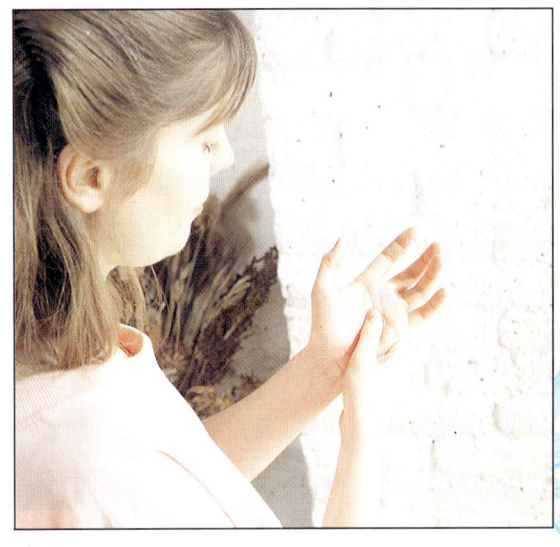

6 Using small circling movements of the thumbs, circle the palm area, applying quite firm pressure. Repeat 5 and 6 on the other side.

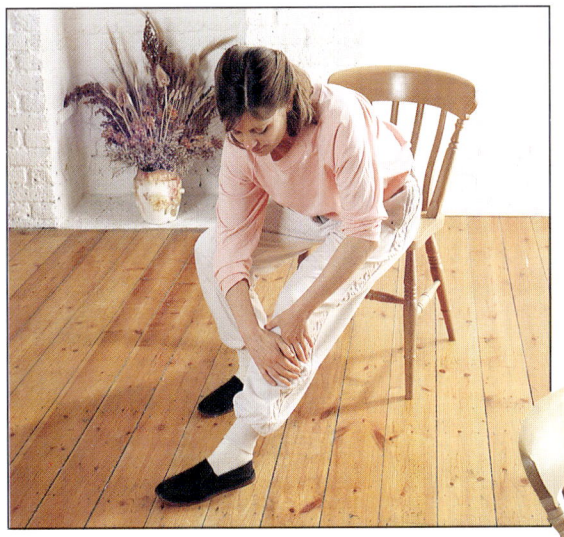

8 Using circular movements of both thumbs, circle the sole of the foot from the heel to toe. Repeat 7 and 8 on the other side.

7 Using the whole hand, scrunch the muscles from the top of the leg right the way down to the ankle and off through the foot.

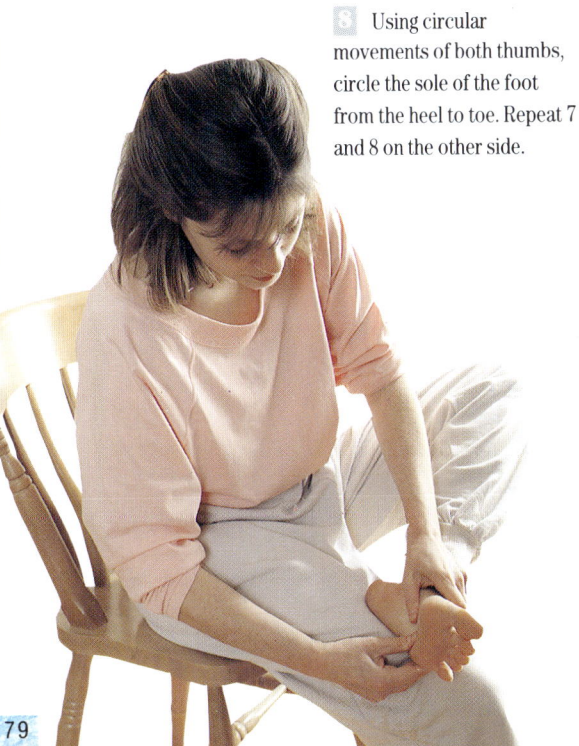

AROMATHERAPY

The use of the essential oils – aromatic chemicals – found in plants, flowers and trees to promote and maintain health, either taken internally or by inhalation. As well as the benefits derived from their smells, many essential oils have important chemical properties: they can be anti-inflammatory, anti-septic or anti-bacterial. Digitalis, for example, is an essential oil from the foxglove that is used in the treatment of heart problems; while the contraceptive pill was developed from the essential oil of the yam. Since they have these properties, some essential oils are poisonous in large doses – digitalis is one of these.

Aromatherapy has been used as a healing technique for thousands of years; the ancient Egyptians, Greeks and Romans all used essential oils to aid relaxation, improve circulation and to help the healing of wounds. The technique spread through the rest of Europe during medieval times, but it declined as the modern pharmaceutical industry developed. However, the art was revived – and the name of 'aromatherapy' was coined – by a French chemist called Gattefossé, who wrote a book on the subject in 1928.

Gattefossé had burnt his hand during an experiment and dipped it into a pot of lavender oil standing nearby. To his surprise the pain disappeared rapidly and the burn healed quickly. He, and others, started to experiment with essential oils, with the result that the effects of many essential oils are known and generally recognized. Today, aromatherapy is practised widely in Europe, where it is frequently combined with other, more mainstream therapies under the direction of a conventional medical doctor.

Because essential oils must be harvested with great care, using specific parts of a plant at set times of the year, or day, they tend to be expensive. Huge quantities of plant material, too, are needed to produce even small quantities of oil – it takes 100 kg of rose petals, for example, to make 0.5 l of rose oil. There is no alternative to this painstaking procedure as another French chemist, Valnet, has shown in the laboratory that substitutes do not have the same effects as the natural oils.

Nevertheless, essential oils can be bought from a wide range of health shops, chemists and beauty parlours. Quality is paramount, though – do not try to skimp on price. Nor should you buy in quantity, since the oils have a short shelf-life, and should be kept away from the light.

Method

Essential oils can be taken at home in two ways: as part of a massage and as an inhalation. A carrier oil is needed for a massage, since the essential oil will be very concentrated, and overuse can cause allergies or skin irritation. The most common carrier oils are soya, grape seed, avocado and almond.

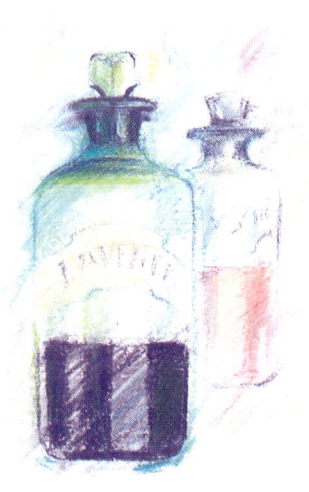

MEDICAL ALERT

Essential oils should never be taken internally except under the direction of a qualified, experienced aromatherapist – some essential oils can be harmful.

1. To make up a massage oil, mix two to three drops of essential oil to 5 ml (1 tsp) of carrier oil. In order for the oil to be absorbed properly, the skin should be absolutely dry and also warm. Take a warm bath and ensure that the room you are using is well heated; in the late evening make sure that everything is prepared in

Selected Stress Symptoms and Their Essential Oils

Use the list of stress symptoms below as a guide, and experiment to find out which oils work best for you. Try one at a time, or make up your own recipes by mixing the different oils that treat the symptom together: four drops of camomile, for example, with four of marjoram and two drops of sandalwood placed in your bath to relieve tension.

Tension – bergamot; camomile; marjoram; neroli; sandalwood; camphor; jasmine.
Colic – marjoram; clary sage; juniper.
Indigestion – bergamot; fennel; lemon; peppermint.
Diarrhoea – eucalyptus; juniper; neroli; sandalwood.
Muscular Aches and Pains – eucalyptus; rosemary; sage.
Depression – bergamot; geranium; jasmine; neroli; rose; ylang ylang.
Insomnia – camphor; camomile; jasmine; marjoram; neroli.
Headaches – cardamon; lavender; marjoram; peppermint; rose.

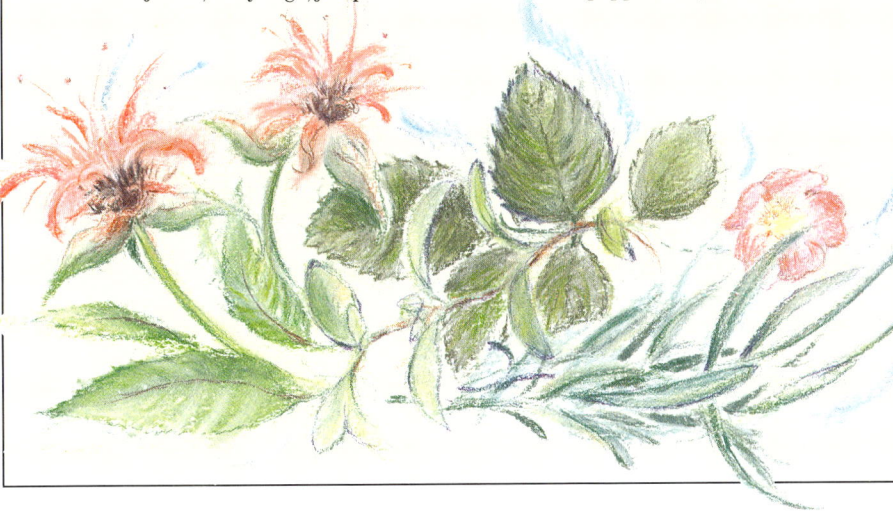

advance, so that you can go to bed straight after the massage – this will increase the effectiveness of it. Use the massage techniques explained under Massage concentrating on any problem areas.

2 If you prefer to take the essential oil as an inhalation, you can use one of two methods: either put 10 drops of essential oil on a handkerchief, and inhale from it deeply; or put 10 drops in a bowl of hot water, cover your head with a towel and breathe in the fumes. For an inhalation or compress place the essential oil directly into the water or onto the compress. One of the best and most relaxing methods of inhaling essential oils, though, is to lie in a warm bath that has been laced with drops of oil, relax and let your skin absorb the oils as you breathe in their perfume. Otherwise, try putting a few drops of oil in a foot bath at the end of a tiring day.

MEDICAL ALERT

Recent research has shown that some essential oils have effects that are not properly understood; these should be avoided. In particular, basil oil appears to cause cancer when taken in large quantities; fennel oil stimulates production of oestrogen, a female hormone, and should not be taken by women who have breast cancer; pennyroyal oil can induce a miscarriage.

SMELL THERAPY

The idea that our sense of smell might have a direct effect upon our perceptions of well-being was considered centuries ago. For example, in his Essay on Smells, written in 1580, Montaigne, the prolific French essayist, suggested that "Physicians might ... make greater use of scents than they do, for I have often noticed that they cause changes in me, and act on my spirits ... which makes me agree with the theory that the introduction of incense and perfume into the churches ... was for the purpose of raising our spirits, and of exciting and purifying our senses, the better to fit us for contemplation".

It is very difficult to explain what the sense of smell is – we know that we capture aromas through sensory receptors in our noses (modern research indicates that we can also absorb smells through the skin), and that the brain recognizes them as either pleasant or unpleasant, but why this distinction should be made is not clear. Everything has a smell, though some things obviously smell more strongly than others. Many animals have a highly developed sense of smell; people, however, have always relied more on sight than on smell for survival

Method

Scents can be categorized into three types, called 'notes' by perfumers, according to the time it takes for them to evaporate. High notes evaporate quickly, but give an instant impact and are stimulating; middle notes are more subtle, tending to be warm or fortifying; and base notes are long-lasting, relaxing and soothing. Most perfumes are manufactured so as to contain elements of all three notes.

1 Use smell in your day-to-day life. First throw away any old perfume as the scent will deteriorate with time. Check the house for any unpleasant smells, such as mustiness or staleness, and open the windows to clear them away. If you or your friends smoke, empty the ashtrays frequently. Make sure strong smelling foods, such as garlic or curry, are kept in air-tight containers, so they do not affect everything else near them.

2 Wear a perfume or aftershave that evokes pleasant memories and thoughts, and favourable reactions in others. Test out different scents – in a department store in the case of commercial perfumes, or in a chemists or health shop for aromatherapy oils and waters (see Aromatherapy). Do not try more than one or two at any one visit, or you will start to confuse the scents. Spray a little onto the inside of your wrist and smell it immediately for the high note, again in an hour for the middle note, and again in about five hours for the base note. Buy several different perfumes or oils so that you have one to fit every mood.

3 Place a few drops of a soothing oil in each room – in a humidifier, an oil vaporizer or a bowl of warm water. Choose the aroma to fit your mood. Or put pot pourri of flowers and herbs in your rooms – but remember to keep them fresh.

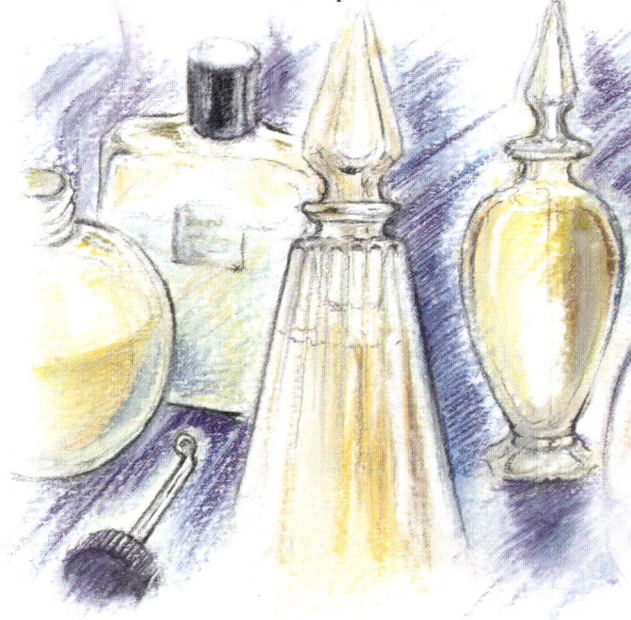

SMELL THERAPY

and as a result our sensitivity to smell is underdeveloped, although this tends to vary from one culture to another. Recently, however, research has shown that smell not only affects our perception of individuals, but has a direct effect on our general mood. This must be partly instinctive, but of course is also due to unconscious associations with past experiences: the antiseptic smell of a hospital, for example, is unnoticed by health workers, but can produce stress many years later in a patient who has unpleasant memories. The perfume worn by one's mother is often remembered throughout one's life, and instantly recognized if worn by someone else, triggering childhood memories. It is an interesting fact that what people consider pleasant and unpleasant in terms of smell varies remarkably little, either through history or across cultural boundaries.

The effect of smell on our moods is now so widely recognized that it is being used commercially to assist sales (one hosiery manufacturer found that sales increased by 25 per cent if their tights were impregnated with a pleasant scent), and in public places to alter or maintain moods: soothing aromas are used in New York's subway stations to induce calm. You too can use a range of different smells to change your mood, reducing stress and increases relaxation.

4 Fresh flowers and plants give off lovely, evocative aromas, so treat yourself to a bouquet of sweet-smelling flowers when you feel low. Be careful if you buy chrysanthemums, though – their water needs to be changed frequently to prevent the woody stems from creating an unpleasant aroma in the water.

5 Perfume your clothes by storing them in drawers with scented liners or sachets of flowers – lavender or rosemary provide just the right degree of subtlety.

6 Try to make sure – tactfully, of course – that your family and work colleagues smell pleasant, and have no problems with personal hygiene.

7 Try placing a few drops of perfume in your bath water before you get in.

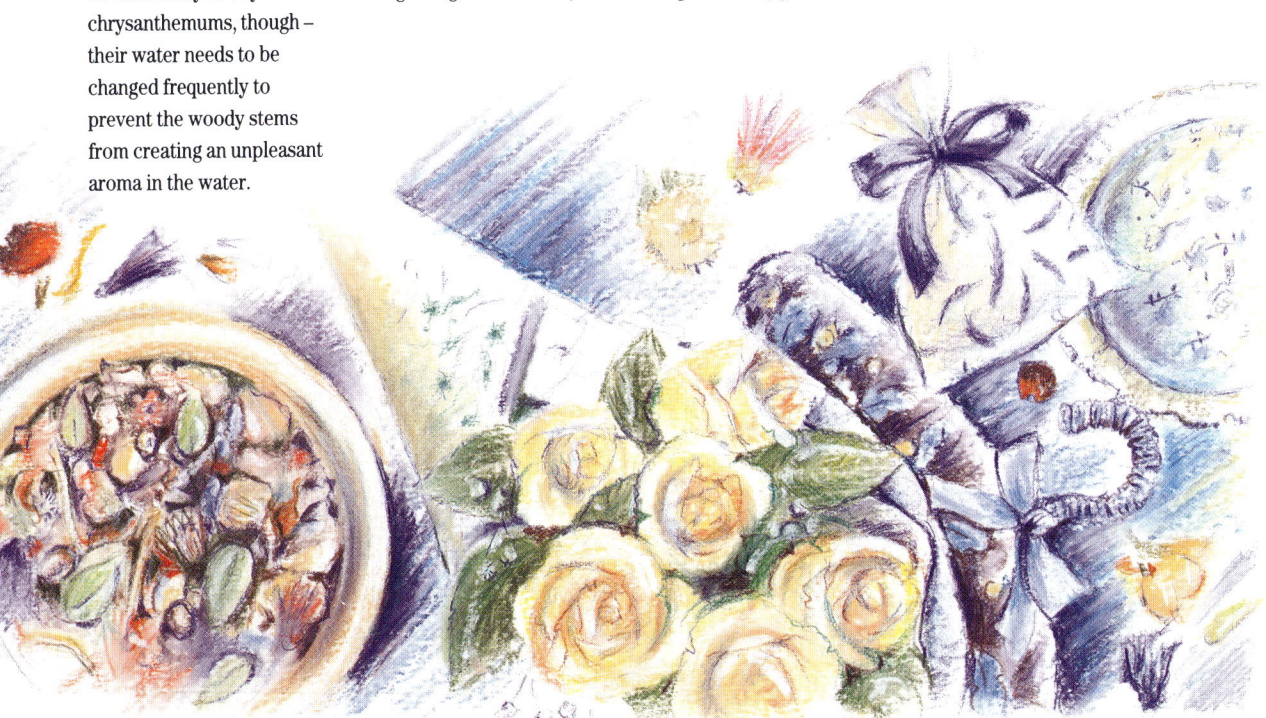

ACUPRESSURE/DO-IN/SHIATSU

Acupressure and shiatsu are like acupuncture without needles. Shiatsu is a Japanese word meaning 'finger pressure'; it was originally the Japanese form of Chinese acupressure, but over time developed characteristics of its own. Both acupressure and shiatsu promote health by restoring the flow of healing energy (chi) along special pathways, named 'meridians' by ancient Chinese healers. These are associated with the vital functions by conducting energy to and from each organ of the body along 12 paired meridian pathways: six cover the legs and lower torso and six cover the arms and upper torso; two further meridians, unpaired, run down the back and front of the torso. The whole system is like an alternative blood circulation, though it cannot yet be identified by anatomists. Acupoints are fixed points on each meridian at the surface of the skin which act as entrances and exits for the vital internal healing force. Sometimes they become blocked, or the flow of healing energy through the meridian becomes sluggish: by exerting finger and thumb pressure upon these points acupressure helps to remove blockages and increase the flow.

Two theories currently help to explain the success of acupressure: first, that pressure on an acupoint restores the natural balance of the body by releasing the body's own pain-killing hormone – endorphin – so relieving many of the symptoms of stress and aiding relaxation. The second, the Gate-Control Theory, starts with the fact that two bundles of nerves transmit messages to the brain from each source – one transmits pain, the other pressure. Messages travelling through pressure nerves travel faster to the brain than those running through pain fibres, and on arrival cause the 'gate' to close, because the brain can only receive so many sensations at once.

Use the illustrations opposite to find acupoints which may help you to relieve some common symptoms of stress. Then experiment to discover your 'tender spots' – these are your personal acupoints, called *ah shi*. They are ofen found around the head and neck – in the centre of the cheeks, for example, the base of the neck, just outside the corners of the eyes and at the centre point between the eyebrows.

Do-In is the self-help version of Acupressure and Shiatsu, which you can practise at home by stimulating the acupoints that feel tender or painful. In Japan, where they view the therapy as a technique for early diagnosis and disease prevention, it continues to be a simple home treatment often practised by members of a family on each other.

Method

Acupressure may be repeated up to five times a day with each session lasting around 20 minutes, though relief is often felt after as little as five minutes.

1. Press down firmly on an acupoint with the ball of the thumb or tips of the fingers, increasing the pressure gradually to a weight of around 5 g (try this out on some kitchen scales).

2. Hold for about 20 seconds and then release slowly and gently.

3. Wait for a further 10 seconds and then repeat up to five times.

4. When you have mastered the basic technique, try making small circular movements in a clockwise direction as you apply pressure.

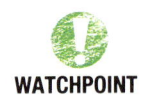

WATCHPOINT

Pressure should be firm, but not produce pain. If there is pain lessen the pressure exerted. Take care not to let your fingernails dig in to the skin – if necessary, cut them.

ACUPRESSURE

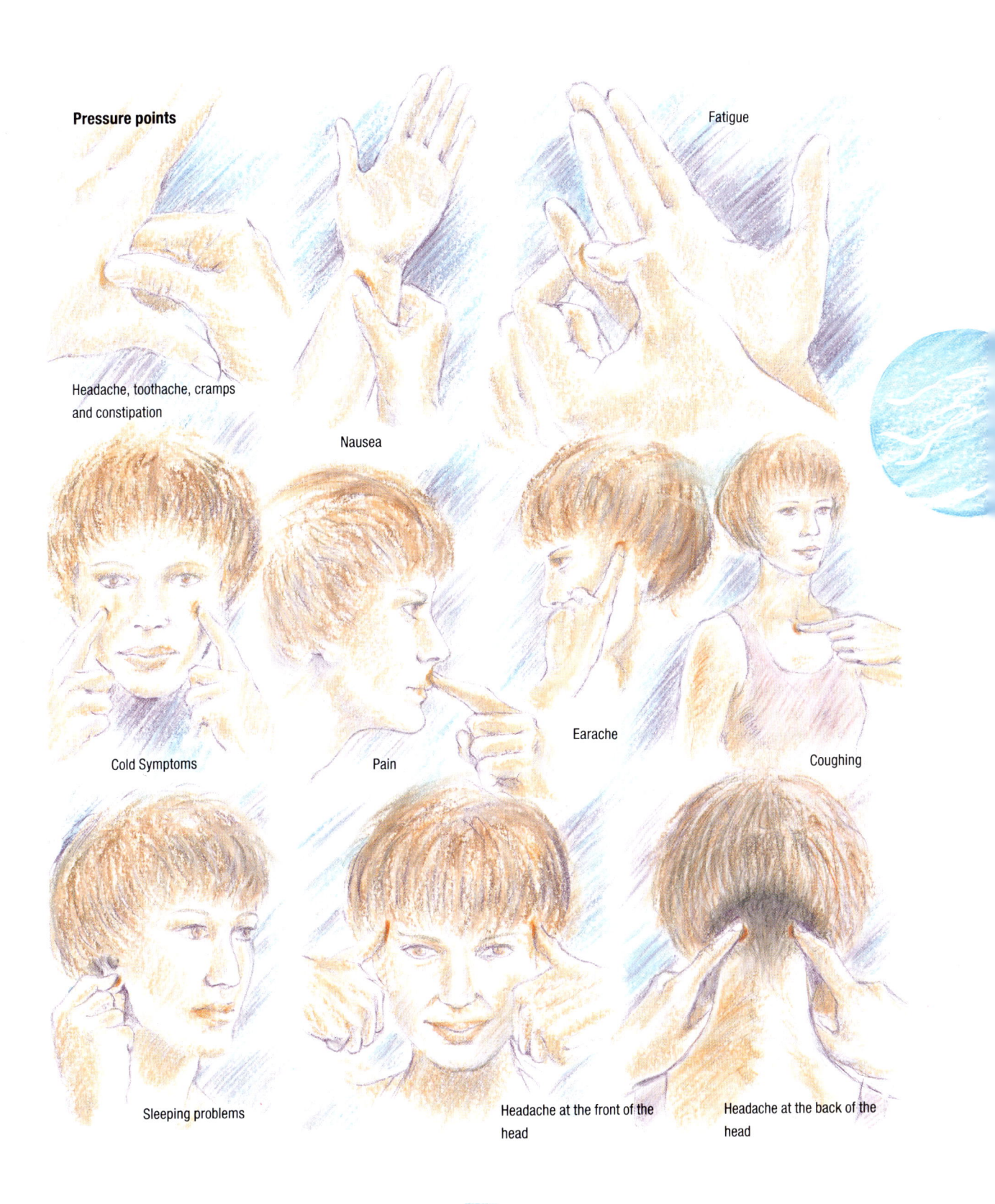

Pressure points

Headache, toothache, cramps and constipation

Nausea

Fatigue

Cold Symptoms

Pain

Earache

Coughing

Sleeping problems

Headache at the front of the head

Headache at the back of the head

TECHNIQUES

REFLEXOLOGY

An ancient Chinese and Egyptian technique that views all illness as the result of blocked energy in the body. Based on the proposition that the organs of the body are mirrored in the feet (and also to a certain extent in the hands), reflexology seeks to detect blocked energy channels by applying pressure to those points where the energy pathways or channels come to the surface. It is held that each channel relates to a zone of the body, to the organs in that zone – the lower back relates to the heel, for example. So, by pressing upon the feet in certain ways, reflexologists can determine which organs are being deprived of energy and restore the balance.

Reflexology was first introduced to the West under the name of zone therapy by Dr William Fitzgerald, an American physician, in the 1920s – though some claim that the technique has always been known and used by native Americans. In the 1930s Fitzgerald's techniques were taken further through the efforts of a nurse called Eunice D Ingham, whose *Stories the Feet Can Tell* was first published in 1932. Both Fitzgerald and Ingham found that firm pressure at particular points on the feet could cause significant effects in other parts of the body. Later, the technique was introduced to Britain by Doreen Bayly, one of Eunice Ingham's students. Since Fitzgerald's first experiments, reflexology has become immensely popular in the Western world. There are now hundreds of reflexologists, many of whom combine the technique with acupressure, homoeopathy and osteopathy.

Reflexologists rely on the sensation of pain indicated by the patient when pressure is applied to a particular part of the foot in order to detect the presence of a problem – the location of the energy blockage and the affected bodily organ depending on which area of the foot and the level of pain when pressed. As such, the technique is diagnostic. It does not, however, attempt to diagnose the nature or cause of the problem – just its location in the body.

Having identified the existence and location of the problem, reflexologists treat it by triggering the body's own healing powers. This is done by deeply massaging the appropriate site on the foot to stimulate and restore the free flow of energy – the 'life force', found in all living things – in 10 zonal pathways. These pathways run straight down the body and come to the surface at the feet, hands and ears. So problems in the right shoulder are reflected in the right foot and hand, and heart conditions can be detected in the left foot and hand. The foot as a whole gives a map of the body, similar to that found in the brain, with the big toe representing the head, the spine running down the centre of the sole of the foot and lower back at the heel (*see diagram*). Three paths run across the foot, reflecting the shoulders, the waist and the hips, making the map complete. When these points are stimulated, waste deposits and congestion in the energy pathways are removed, improving blood circulation and gland function. The overall effect is to relax the whole system, thus reflexology can be particulary useful in the treatment of stress-related problems. Though the technique is at its most effective in the hands of a reflexologist, the methods demonstrated on these pages can be used as a self-help treatment – at home, ideally, but anywhere in a pinch. The help of a friend or partner would be useful.

WATCHPOINT

The reflex point for the solar plexus (in the centre of the torso) is especially useful when trying to increase relaxation and treat stress, so should be treated at each session (*see diagram*). The sensation of 'butterflies in the stomach' comes from the solar plexus.

Parts of the body reflected in different points on the soles of the feet

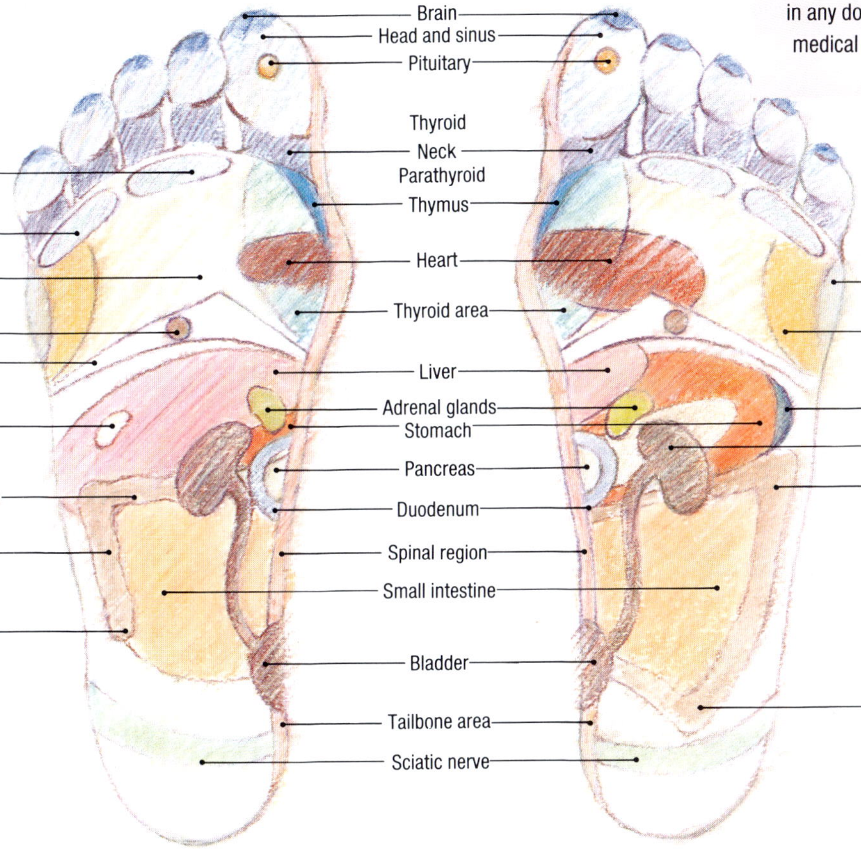
Brain
Head and sinus
Pituitary
Thyroid
Neck
Parathyroid
Thymus
Eyes
Ears
Lung
Heart
Arm
Solar plexus
Diaphragm
Thyroid area
Shoulder
Liver
Gallbladder
Adrenal glands
Stomach
Spleen
Kidney
Pancreas
Transverse colon
Duodenum
Descending colon
Ascending colon
Spinal region
Small intestine
Ileocecal valve
Bladder
Sigmoid colon
Tailbone area
Sciatic nerve

Right sole

Left sole

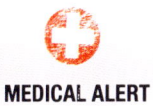

MEDICAL ALERT

Some practitioners believe that treatment should not be attempted during pregnancy, or if you have heart problems, thrombosis or shingles. If in any doubt, ask your medical practitioner.

Method

Use the charts to find the reflex points where you should apply pressure to detect a problem. The most sensitive reflex points are on the feet, so these are explained here. You can also obtain charts for the hands.

1 First wash and dry your feet. Make yourself as comfortable as possible, being careful not to strain your back. If possible, lay your foot across your lap.

2 Always start by giving the whole foot – both sole, ankle and top – a thorough massage. Use talcum powder or a relaxing aromatherapy oil to help the

TECHNIQUES

hands glide smoothly over the skin. Make sure that the foot is relaxed and held loosely and that it is your hands that are doing the work.

3 Move all the joints in the foot and ankle in turn. Start with the ankle and make a circling movement, first in one direction and then the other. Move the foot up and down and in and out.

4 Take each toe in turn, starting with the big toe, and bend it backwards and forwards and from side to side, then grasp each toe firmly and pull gently as though to lengthen it slightly. Squeeze gently on the web between each toe as you move from toe to toe.

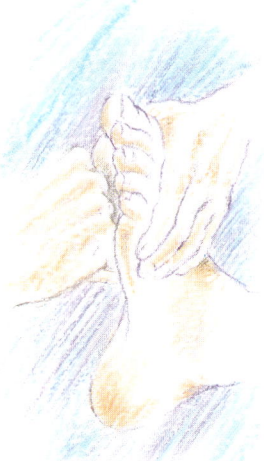

5 Next, massage the whole foot – paying particular attention to the sole of the foot using the massage techniques of effleurage and pettrisage (see p72). You may find it easier to massage the soles of your feet by making your hand into a fist.

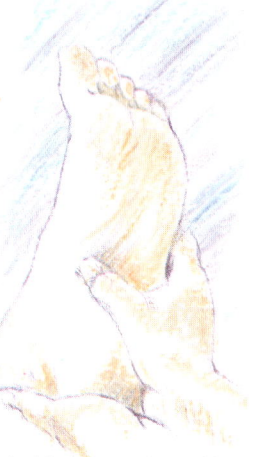

6 When the foot feels loose and relaxed start to knead all the reflex points in turn with your thumb. Be careful not to dig your thumb nail into the skin – if necessary cut the nail. There are two main ways to check the reflex points: the first is a firm downward pressure with the end and the side of the thumb at a fixed point for about 30 seconds, followed by a slight rotational movement, whilst maintaining the pressure, for another 30 seconds; the second is a 'creeping' or 'walking' movement with thumb or finger – push down steadily with either and, maintaining the pressure, 'walk' it by moving the wrist up and down. This can be difficult at first, but usually becomes second nature with time and practice.

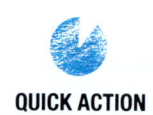

Moving the foot up and down

Massaging the sole of the foot

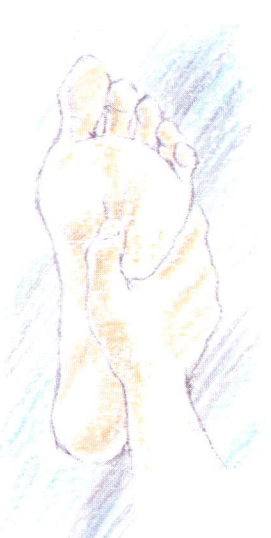

Applying pressure to sensitive points

Bending the toes backwards and forwards

Finding the reflex points

QUICK ACTION

Once you have identified the tender points on your feet, you will be able to use reflexology at work, on a journey or in the kitchen waiting for the kettle to boil! A few minutes of deep pressure can help reduce the symptoms of stress or prevent their onset – especially if you always remember to treat the reflex point for the solar plexus. Remember, too, that you can always massage your foot through a stocking or a sock if necessary.

As a preventive measure, massage the relevant reflex points for any symptoms you are prone to even if no pain is felt at the time.

7 Feel for any tender or sensitive reflex points and check for any grit-like nodules under the skin. These are often found at reflex points in which there is a blockage in the corresponding energy pathway.

8 Once the whole foot has been covered and any tender points noted, concentrate treatment on those areas, using the same techniques. It is normal to feel some pain while doing this, especially where there are nodules, but you should not give such deep pressure that the pain is excruciating. Under a steady pressure the nodules will break up like lumps of sugar. Treat each area for approximately four minutes during each session.

9 Repeat the procedure on the other foot.

METAMORPHIC THERAPY

Robert St John, a reflexologist, developed the metamorphic technique in the 1960s following the oriental principle that areas of the feet correspond to the period spent in the mother's womb between conception to birth. He believed that all our emotional as well as our physical and mental patterns and responses are formed during the gestation period. According to the theory, energy blocks that occurred in the womb can be released by massaging the spinal reflexes of the feet and hands. The treatment is similar to that of reflexology and starts with a general foot massage. In the case of the foot, concentrate on the central line down the sole and the arch of the foot. For the hand, use the outside edge running down the thumb and the back of the wrist. The metamorphic technique also treats reflex points at the back of the head – the line down the centre of the head to the nape of the neck and back up each side to behind the ears.

Relaxation Aids

A number of specialist foot massage aids are available, all of which help general relaxation – they can be used either at home or at work, where even just a few minutes massage will help. Alternatively, roll a golf ball around the sole of the foot against the floor, or use the palms of your hands; a rolling pin, too, can be used to massage the soles of the feet, as can a bar or cross-piece beneath a table. Some people find it comfortable and relaxing to wear wooden-soled, contoured shoes or sandals. Or you can try walking around as much as possible in bare feet. This not only helps to counteract any stresses put on the feet whilst wearing shoes, especially high-heels, but also heightens the sensations that the foot receives and transmits to the brain. This aids balance, relaxation and good posture.

WATCHPOINT

If considerable pain that does not disappear momentarily is felt at any particular point, stop your own treatment and consult a professional reflexologist.

WATCHPOINT

Metamorphic therapists feel that treatment should not be given for longer than one hour a week, because it is better to release these deep-seated blockages slowly. Sometimes the hour is split up into several even shorter sessions.

TECHNIQUES

HYDROTHERAPY

A belief in the healing properties of water goes back at least to the classical civilizations of ancient Greece and Rome, but was probably held for many centuries before them. The Greeks believed that water possessed all the properties necessary for healing and maintaining health, and the Romans took this idea a step further by integrating hydrotherapy into their social life, building temples and baths near to natural springs. People would gather in them to relax, chatter and have ailments of all types treated; many such centres also had gymnasiums, massage tables and libraries – in fact they were the forerunner of today's health farms and spas.

Today there is a resurgence of interest in hydrotherapy, since it can help a number of problems, and in particular those caused by stress. We all know and appreciate the relaxation and feeling of well-being that follows a hot, peaceful, sweet-smelling bath. Swimming, too, is an excellent and relaxing form of exercise.

One earlier renewal of interest in hydrotherapy, at the turn of the 19th century, could hardly be said to have relaxation in mind. Vincent Priessnitz, an Austrian, had a fervent belief in the healing properties of plain, cold water, and opened a spa at Grafenberg (now in Czechoslovakia) to put his ideas into practice. Patients flocked to the spa to endure a series of spartan and rigorous treatments. These included cold compresses, rubs with wet sheets, cold plunge-baths and walking with bare feet on the morning dew. As Priessnitz's popularity increased, so his treatments became harsher – buckets of cold water were thrown down on patients from such a height and with such force that a bar was provided for their support.

But Father Sebastian Kneip (1821–1897) from Worshofen, Bavaria, was the true father of modern-day hydrotherapy in Germany, where the technique is especially popular. He believed in Priessnitz's

▶
■ Swimming is a great form of exercise, suitable for all ages. Keep a note of the opening times of local pools – they may be open early and late.

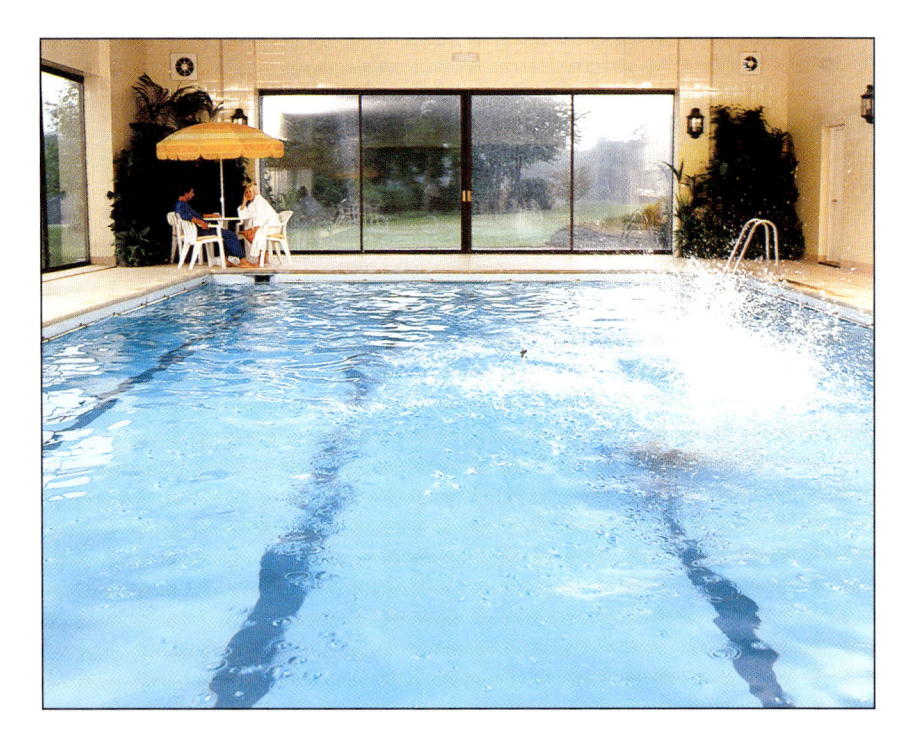

treatments, but was much more gentle – though he still expected his patients to walk bare-foot in the snow and wade in cold streams. Kneip's ideas spread quickly through Europe and spas sprang up wherever natural spring water was available. Unfortunately, many of them were run by charlatans, and hydrotherapy was scorned by the medical profession of the time as unorthodox and dangerous – in one medical journal of the time, hydrotherapy was indexed under water-death.

· In over-enthusiastic hands hydrotherapy could indeed be fatal. In 1796, Robert Burns, the famous Scottish poet, took a water cure for his acute rheumatism – probably the result of his work as a customs officer in the rain-swept western Highlands of Scotland. The treatment prescribed was to stand in the freezing estuary waters of the Solway Firth up to his armpits for two hours each day – he died a few months later.

Today, however, hydrotherapy is used in a more sensible way, and is fully recognized to be of benefit by the medical profession; in fact, it is used in many treatments given by physiotherapists for a wide range of complaints. In Britain and America, treatment tends to be confined to health farms and specialist medical centres, but in Europe it is widely used and available to all. In Germany, for example, many people book into a spa for a fortnight each year – their treatment being paid for through medical insurance schemes.

But what does water actually do to help physical problems? For our purposes – reducing stress and aiding relaxation – water is primarily of use in helping to relieve muscular tension. Some people, though, believe that water may, itself, have healing properties since it could retain the 'imprint' of beneficial substances over which it has passed – in the same way as homoeopathic (p138) and Bach Flower Remedies (p141). This, however, is difficult to evaluate in any convincing way.

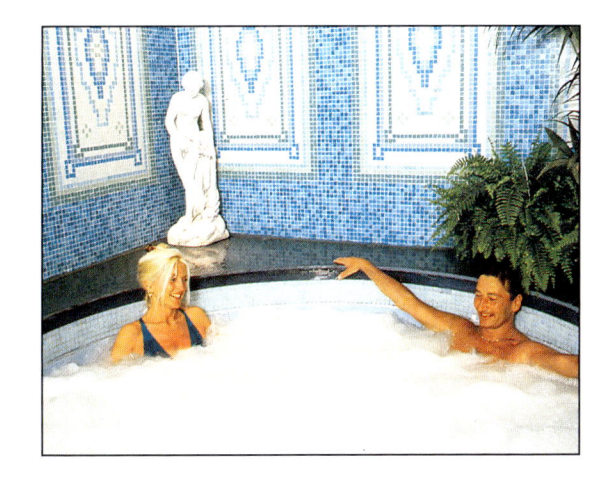

Method
Swimming
Water supports the body, taking part of its weight, so the muscles do not have to strain constantly to maintain a poor posture or position, and can function freely and easily. This makes swimming an excellent way to ease tense muscles and relieve joint stiffness. Swim hard to get rid of aggression, or laze along to banish tiredness and anxiety. Float, close your eyes, and feel the water ripple over the skin; relish the freedom of movement and imagine all the tension draining out of your body and into the water.

Jacuzzis & Showering
If you are lucky enough to have access to a jacuzzi, relax into it and allow the bubbles and jets of water to pummel your muscles. Aim the jets at any particularly tense ones, especially those in the shoulders and neck. A jacuzzi is ideal for this, but you can achieve a similar effect with a shower. Turn the shower up to its maximum strength, at a comfortable temperature, and focus its jets onto tense muscles; feel the water pouring down your body and draining away, and imagine your problems and tension going the same way. If you have a hand-held shower, turn it full on and hold it under the bath water near the skin. Massage the muscles, feel the skin rippling and the tension oozing away.

▲ Sitting in a jacuzzi is a very relaxing experience – try and find out if there is a club near you with these facilities.

TECHNIQUES

Salt rub

Rub yourself vigorously all over with normal kitchen salt and a little body oil. Rinse off under a warm shower and rub some more body oil into the skin. This aids the circulation, helps to eliminate toxins from the skin and leaves it feeling smooth, supple and glowing.

Saunas & Turkish baths

Both of these help rid the skin of toxins and improve the circulation. At home a shower that is alternately hot and cold can have much the same effect. Some people recommend going straight to bed after the cold shower – this is very invigorating, yet makes sleep deep and relaxing.

Sitz bath

Sit in your bath with cold water up to your hips, but with your feet in a washing-up bowl full of warm water. Stay there for 10 minutes, then reverse the process – put cold water in the bowl, and warm water in the bath. Stay for 10 minutes, then run through the procedure again. Used three times a week, a sitz bath will help the circulation and relieve tired legs and feet as well as aching muscles.

Bathing

Soak in a deep, hot bath. Pamper yourself with bath oils (see 'Aromatherapy' p80), bubbles, colour (see 'Colour Therapy' p142), relax, let your legs and arms float, feel weightless, close your eyes and imagine a beautiful beach scene (see 'Visualization' p122) – let the tensions of the day seep out of your body and float away. Have a large, warm towel ready to step into; cosset yourself, fall into a deep, comfortable chair or your bed and relax.

Epsom salts bath

Epsom Salts are, in fact, a chemical compound called magnesium sulphate, which induces sweating. For an average bath you need approximately 5 lb (just over 2 kg) of commercial magnesium sulphate (obtainable from health food shops and large chemists). Put the Epsom Salts in your bath, and run the water as hot as you can stand it – though not, of course, at a temperature that would scald. Lie in the bath for at least 15 minutes and top up with hot water when necessary, so that you keep up a good sweat. Finish off with a shower and then rub yourself down vigorously with warm towels. Epsom Salts baths were first used in World War I to treat shell-shocked soldiers; they were found to calm the nerves, improve the circulation, rid the skin of toxins and help to heal a number of skin conditions.

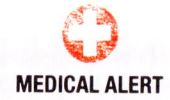

FLOATATION TANK

The use of floatation tanks is a fairly recent innovation, and is only available at a few specialist health centres. The treatment starts with a thorough wash of the body and the hair, to clean off any dirt and excess body oil. The patient then lies down in a tank containing a concentrated solution of Epsom Salts – enough to cover the body – in a warm, dark, sound-proof room. The Salts increase the buoyancy of the water, and help prevent the skin from crinkling. The patient stays in the tank for at least 45 minutes and preferably around two hours. In the silence and the dark, with a feeling of weightlessness, tensions and stresses float away, leaving a sense of total physical and mental well-being. It is claimed that the treatment works by stimulating the production of the body's natural pain-relieving hormones – the endorphins – to ease pain, by lowering blood pressure and by reducing the levels of stress-related biochemicals in the body.

MEDICAL ALERT

Epsom Salts can exacerbate some skin conditions. Before you attempt a full Epsom Salts bath, apply them to a small area of skin and wait for 24 hours to test your response – or ask your family doctor.

HYDROTHERAPY EXERCISES

For relaxation
- Teach yourself to float. Your toes should just be sticking out of the water, with your body in a straight line – do not let your hips droop, as this will pull the rest of the body down and you will sink. Your head should be slightly back, with the water just lapping on your forehead – do not tuck your chin in. Relax completely and let the buoyancy of the water take your weight. Breathe evenly and deeply and empty your mind – concentrate on the feeling of the water lapping around your body.

Floating is not as easy as it sounds and quite a bit of practice is needed to perfect the technique, especially in a swimming pool; if possible, practise in the sea, where the salt in the water increases buoyancy. If you find floating impossible borrow or buy some floats.

- Swim slowly and gently, alternating between your back and front. Use the strokes that are easiest for you. Maintain a steady rhythm and concentrate on the feel of the water flowing past you. Many swimming pools have time and space put aside for those who want to do laps. This is an excellent time to swim for relaxation, since you do not have to worry about where other people are in the water.

For fitness
- Swimming is an excellent way of improving overall fitness without causing any damage to the body – as physical fitness increases, relaxation becomes easier and deeper.
- Join a swimming aerobics class.
- Swim laps, starting slowly and gradually increasing the number of laps you swim each day, and, if you wish, the pace at which you swim them.
- Join a swimming club – perhaps take up water polo.

For stiffness and odd aches and pains
All your movements should be slow and steady. Do not force any movement beyond what feels comfortable. Repeat each movement ten times.

- **For your hips and legs** Stand in the pool with water at the level of your chest, holding onto the side of the pool. Swing your legs backwards and forwards, from side to side and in a circular movement.

- **For your shoulders** Kneel in the water at a depth at which the water reaches your neck. Hold onto the side of the pool. Swing your arms alternately backward and forward, side to side and in a circular motion. Shrug your shoulders up and down and round and round.

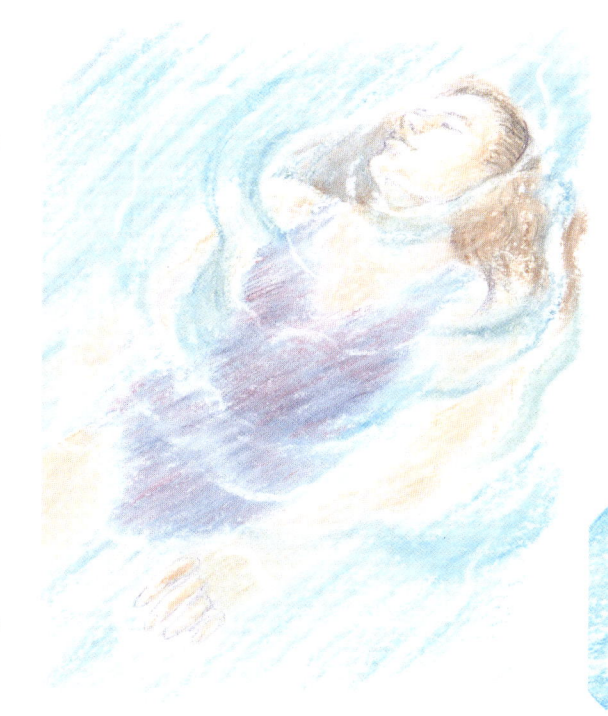

- **For your back** Swim on your back slowly and rhythmically – if necessary, hold a float to your chest. Tuck your chin in slightly, so that you can see your toes as they break the surface – there should not be any heavy splashing. Next, hold onto the side in deep water and curl up and stretch out very slowly, keeping your legs relaxed.

WATCHPOINT

Try to swim regularly for maximum benefit: two or three times a week. Avoid breaststroke if you suffer from neck pains, especially if you are inclined to swim with your head sticking out of the water.

TECHNIQUES

NEGATIVE ION OR AIR IONIZATION THERAPY

MEDICAL ALERT

No adverse side-effects have yet been reported in connection with air ionization therapy – provided that the machine is in good working order. It is therefore important to have yearly maintenance checks carried out on your ionizer, especially if it is in continuous use.

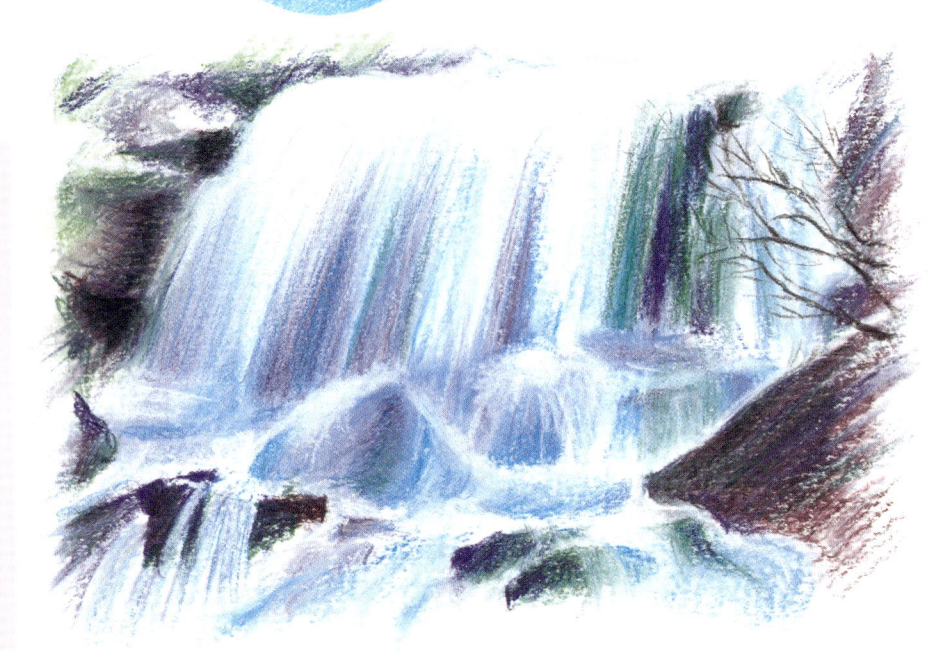

The air that we breathe contains electrically charged particles called ions that either carry a positive or a negative charge. Ions are necessary for good health, but they should be in balance or negatively charged. Positively charged ions, it has been found, endanger health and, according to some therapists, cause people to become sick, tired and emotional.

How many of these ions are in the air varies from one region to another, and the number that are either positively or negatively charged varies too. The atmosphere in mountain and rural areas contains a healthier proportion of negative ions, but these days most people live in towns and cities where negative ions are in short supply – eliminated by smoke, dust and fumes. Many of us work in large office buildings where central heating and air-conditioning systems actually remove negative ions from the air.

Negative Ion therapy aims to prevent disease and counteract particular disorders by replacing these lost ions through the use of special machines called 'ionizers' which can artificially produce negatively charged ions. In this way, the stale, smoky air of a city boardroom can be negatively recharged to the purity of a mountain environment.

At the turn of the century, when the presence of ions in the air was discovered, research was carried out in a number of countries – especially Germany, Britain and Israel – into the effects that ions might have on people. It was discovered that air rich with positive ions affected mood and mental stability, causing irritability, anxiety, headaches, unease and an inability to concentrate. In nature, many of the warm, dry winds that sweep across certain countries, such as the *Foehn* in Switzerland or the *Sharav* in Israel, have the reputation of having an adverse effect on people, causing ill health, for example, general malaise and an increase in the crime rate. Such winds have been found to be rich in positive ions, but it was also found that if people who were suffering from the malaise they caused breathed air rich in negative ions the symptoms disappeared.

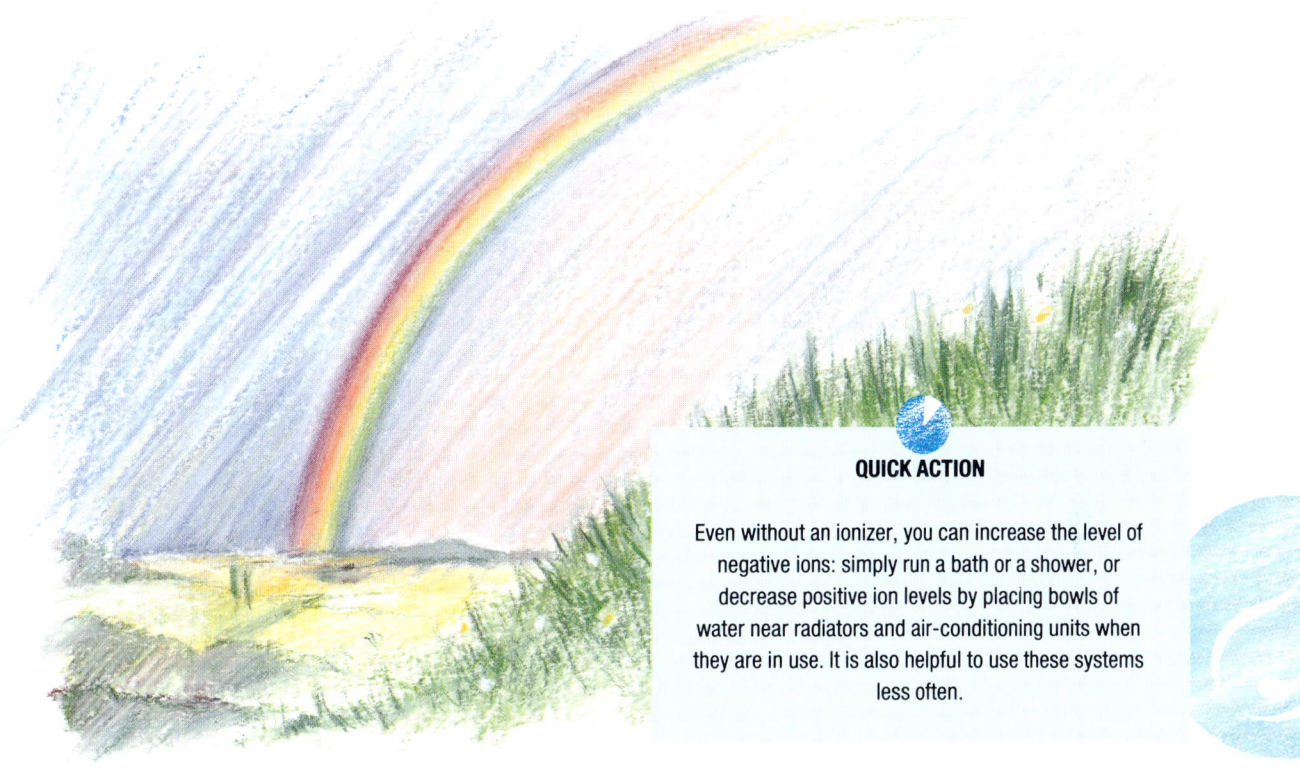

As science has advanced, it has become fairly easy to test the concentration of ions in the air, and such tests have shown that many of the places that have a reputation for being 'healthy' have a naturally high concentration of negative ions in the surrounding air; negative ions seem to induce a general feeling of health and well-being. Linked to this is the fact that more negative ions are formed in the air around running water – waterfalls, downpours and showers, for example. Before a storm, too, many people feel lethargic, irritable and depressed, but afterwards invigorated and cheerful; this may be because the atmosphere is charged with positive ions before a storm, but afterwards contains many more negative ions.

Negative Ion therapy uses the properties of these negatively charged particles – they also include the ability to remove pollutants, such as cigarette smoke, from the air – to treat certain medical conditions, and has had considerable success in ameliorating eczema, burns, depression, headaches and lung problems.

Following a trial with 3,000 patients in a Cologne clinic, it was reported that over 50 per cent obtained total relief from symptoms.

Method

Air ionizers are available from specialist shops or from health centres in various models and sizes, the commonest resembling a small transistor radio. Most models are portable and can be installed in cars, or bedrooms; for example, to treat respiratory disorders an ionizer can be placed on a bedside table. Larger versions are suitable for open-plan living areas, offices, meeting halls, for example. The largest veterans' hospital in the US has an ionizer in each of its recovery rooms.

QUICK ACTION

Even without an ionizer, you can increase the level of negative ions: simply run a bath or a shower, or decrease positive ion levels by placing bowls of water near radiators and air-conditioning units when they are in use. It is also helpful to use these systems less often.

TECHNIQUES

TENS THERAPY

Transcutaneous Electrical Nerve Stimulation, or TENS therapy, for short, makes use of electricity to relieve pain. The potential of electricity as a treatment has been known for thousands of years – early doctors tried to use electric eels in their therapies – but its benefits were limited until the 19th century, when physicists discovered how it could be generated and harnessed. Then electrical treatment became a fad, often used by charlatans in an attempt to cure everything and anything.

In the 1960s, however, the Gate Control Theory of pain relief became generally accepted (*see* Acupressure), and subsequently the TENS machine was produced. This is a small electrical apparatus with electrodes – either two or four – that are placed on the skin. A jelly-like substance is placed under the electrodes to act as a conductor; this allows the electrical current to pass easily through the skin. Not only does the mild electrical stimulation that it gives increase sensory nerve outputs, so as effectively to block the passage of the pain sensations, it also stimulates the body to produce its own pain relieving hormones – the endorphins; this means that pain relief continues for some time after the machine is turned off.

Method

A doctor's prescription is not needed for a TENS machine, which can be bought on the open market. TENS therapy is a useful aid to relaxation in conditions that also cause pain: headaches, for example, menstrual pains, muscular aches, back and neck pains and joint pain. The machine is simple to use and perfectly safe: just follow the manufacturer's instructions.

Place the electrodes over the painful areas, and turn the machine on. Next increase the intensity of stimulation until you feel a pleasant tingling sensation; if you feel any pain, turn the intensity down. The treatment is normally continued for about 30 minutes, but you can use the machine for anything from five minutes to an hour, as often as you like.

Pain relief is normally most effective when the electrodes are placed directly over the most painful spot. Sometimes the effect can last for days, and often the pain disappears for good after a few treatments. Other, more intractable pains may never disappear completely, but there will nearly always be a reduction in the level of pain felt.

MEDICAL ALERT

It is advisable not to use the TENS machine near your eyes, if you have a heart problem or you are pregnant, unless specifically advised to do so by a doctor.

ULTRASOUND

SOUND THERAPY

The use of sound waves to heal. Sound comprises vibrations of variable frequency – human beings can only hear the middle-frequency ranges, while high frequencies are said to be ultrasonic and low frequencies are called infrasonic.

The efficacy of sound therapy relies on the fact that every cell in the human body vibrates at a certain frequency. In health, cells vibrate at their own correct and constant rate. When there is disease for any reason, whether mental or physical, the vibration of effected cells changes to an unnatural rate and rhythm.

Sound therapists believe that by introducing sound waves of the appropriate frequency they can bring the vibrations of such cells back to normal. There is little scientific evidence to support this; however, treatment by sound has been found to be very effective in conventional medicine, working in a different way – either by using the destructive properties of sound to break down tissues, or by using the varying abilities of different types of tissue to absorb or reflect sound waves as a diagnostic tool. The use of the ultrasonic scanner for diagnosis is an example of the latter; the use of sound waves to break up kidney stones is an example of the former. The disintegration properties of sound waves are also utilized in physiotherapy, in the treatment of muscular aches and pains, an excess of scar tissue, and of bruises and inflammation of the joints.

Method

It is now possible to buy an ultrasonic machine for home use, which is similar to the type used by physiotherapists. Such machines play back a magnetic tape on which sound waves of a pre-set depth and range have been recorded – these sound waves break down tissue adhesions and reduce inflammation. As a result ultrasonic machines can be of great help in healing sprains, stiffness and swelling.

This means that ultrasound can also be used to treat the muscular aches and pains that can so often be a sign of stress – although the treatment may not not have any effect on the root cause of the stress.

MEDICAL ALERT

Ultrasound should not, however, be used if you are pregnant, if you have any type of cancer, phlebitis or are in the active stage of rheumatiod arthritis.

TECHNIQUES

T'AI CHI CHUAN

T'ai chi chuan – T'ai chi for short – is an ancient Chinese technique that applies the principles of Taoist philosphy to the art of movement. The basis of Taoist philosophy is the search for natural balance and harmony in all things. It is based on the principle of the yin and the yang (*see* p101), and the idea that to find a personal harmony we need to accept what is – the natural order of the universe – and use this, rather than resisting it, to achieve our goals. In this way we remain in balance both within ourselves and with the outside world. T'ai chi has been described as 'meditation in motion'; each movement or exercise has a symbolic interpretation placed upon the psychological element involved. It aims to expand our consciousness of ourselves as a mental and physical whole and realize the power that we have within us.

The technique is known to have been practised since the 16th century, though there is a legend that it was developed by a Taoist monk called Chang San-Feng in the 12th century. 'T'ai' is the Chinese word for a pole – a strong rod, or centre point. This pole is the dividing line between life's opposites (the yin and yang), as in heat and cold, light and dark and strength and weakness. 'Chi' is our energy force or life force, and Taoists believe that once we can focus on and release this force within us we can use it to combat stress and disease, and so achieve a balanced and relaxed mind and body.

The flowing forms of T'ai chi encourage people to relax and so are particularly helpful in reducing stress and anxiety. The different postures have evocative names.

Push

Press

Lifting hands

Shoulder stroke

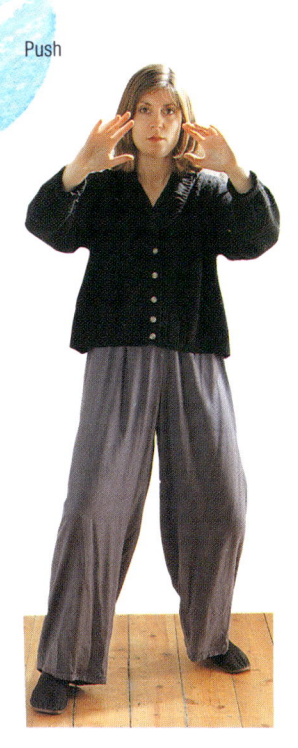

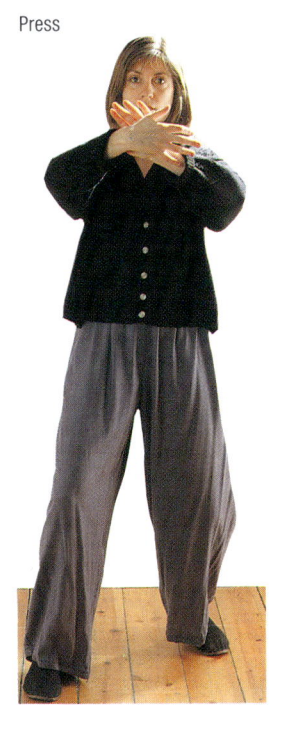

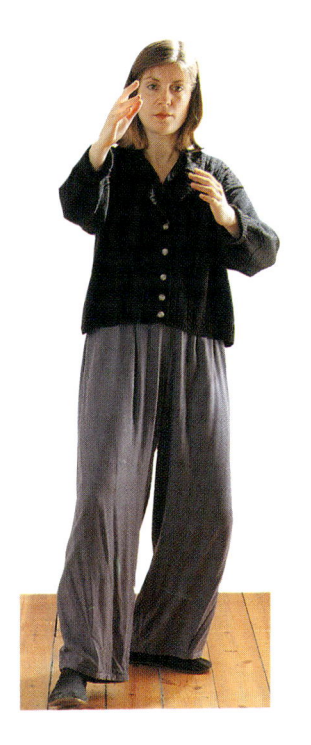

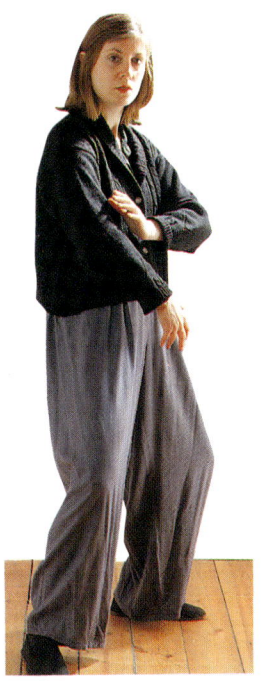

Chang San-Feng is said to have adapted the exercises performed by the monks as an antidote to the many hours spent in meditation, and the martial art known as Chuan, into a series of positions that flow into one another, in which the muscles are kept as relaxed as possible. This mobilizes the chi to utilize external forces and situations to increase our strength, rather than oppose them.

Method

T'ai chi consists of a number of basic postures, called 'forms', and a large and various collection of exercises. Each form is a complicated series of postures that are all linked to give one flowing movement. All the movements are circular and aim to develop muscular control, rather than muscular bulk. In order to learn these, it is best to attend a few classes and then to practise them at home.

Use the examples given on these pages to get a feel for the type of movements in the technique and then experiment by making up some of your own. Keep in mind the main principles, though – especially that the whole body is involved in each movement, not just the part that is moving. After a while the body will become more relaxed; the mind will become relaxed, too, as it concentrates on the flow of relaxed movements.

Ideally T'ai chi should be practised on grass in the open air, but this is not essential. The emphasis is on relaxation, balance and focused tranquillity – no great strength or exertion is required from the student.

Start each movement with the feet placed slightly

Golden rooster stands on one leg

Kick with heel

Step forward to the seven stars

Sweep lotus with leg

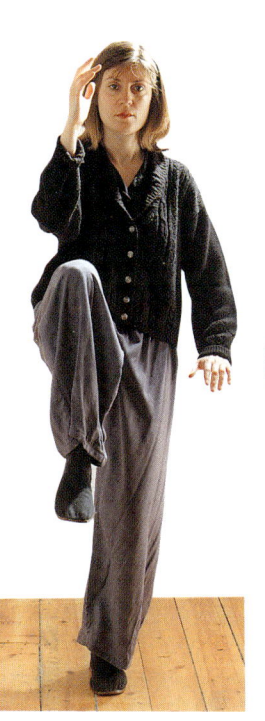

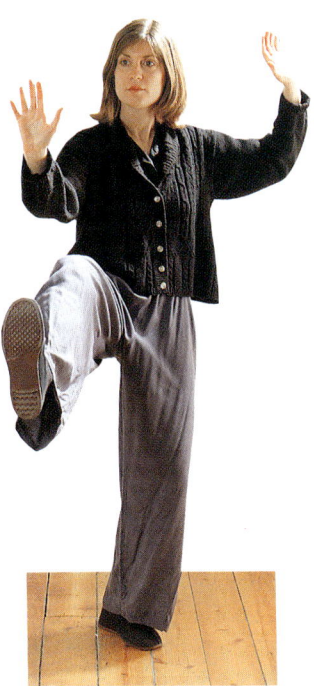

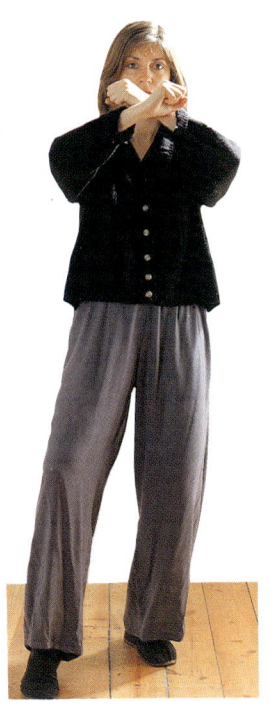

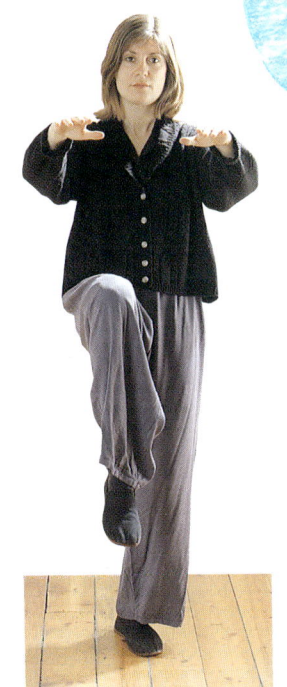

wider apart than the hips – they should feel stuck to the ground. Try to feel the pull of gravity from the ground. Bend the knees slightly and keep the body relaxed and centred. Let your arms hang freely by your side – they should feel long and heavy. Keep your head straight and up – as though a piece of thread is pulling the crown of your head up to the sky.

Work through each movement very slowly, making sure that there is no pain or pulling in the muscles or joints. Keep your muscles as relaxed and as long as possible throughout the movements – never hold them. If you feel tension – in the neck and shoulder muscles, for example – focus your mind on it, but do not try and relax it. Just accept the tension and complete the movement. Take the starting posture again and feel your arms becoming longer and heavier, your chest broader, your back longer and your head higher. Never stop a movement halfway through, even if it feels wrong – complete and start again.

Start each movement at the feet – the stable point – and feel it spread up the legs, through the spine, down the arms and into the centres of the hands, while these make circular or pushing gestures and the breathing is relaxed and deep.

MOVEMENTS

Remember – throughout each exercise the body should be relaxed, the movements slow and the mind centred inwards to feel the flow of energy. Try to forget the presence of time.

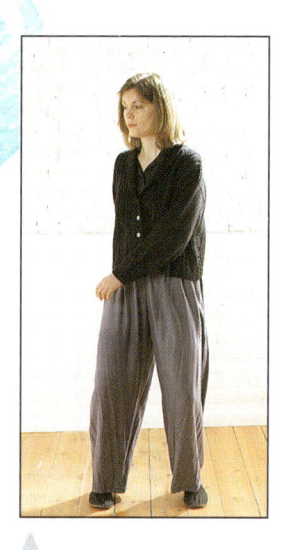

▲ Try the simple warm-up exercises above and on the opposite page. To progress to the postures on the previous page you should find a qualified teacher who will be able to help you maintain correct body alignment as you work – checking, for example, that the spine is straight. Your teacher should also help you to become aware of the spiritual and mental benefits.

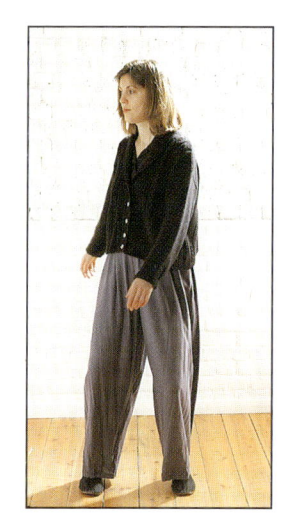

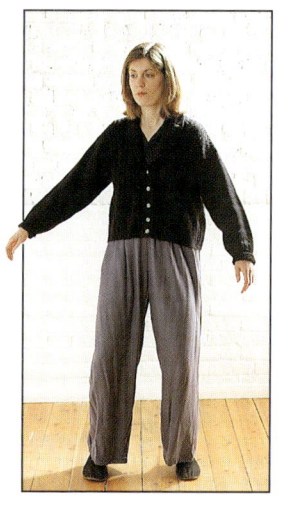

For this exercise stand with your feet parallel and placed slightly wider apart than your hips. Swing your arms slowly and gently from side to side keeping your shoulders level and turning your body as you do so. Don't move your feet and don't force your body to turn more than feels comfortable. Try to relax, clear your mind and let your movements flow.

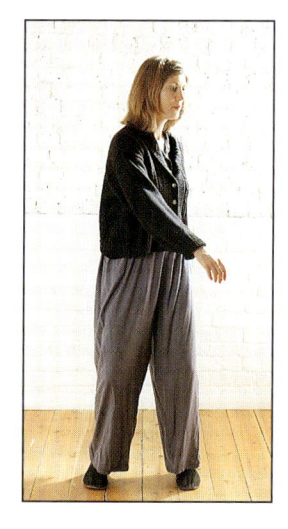

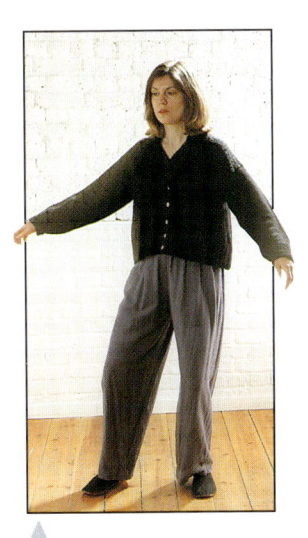

▲ Perform the same exercise as on the previous page but allow your right foot to turn out as you swing right and your left foot to turn out as you swing left. This will allow your body to turn more as your arms swing to each side.

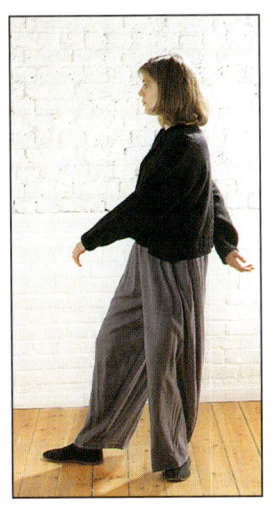

YIN AND YANG

According to ancient Chinese philosophy, good health depends on the maintenance of a balance between two opposing forces – yin and yang. Yin is the dark, passive, feminine principle, representing the interior of the body and solid organs, such as the liver; yang is the light, active, male principle, representing the exterior of the body and hollow organs, such as the heart. Chinese healers believe that anything that upsets the balance between the two, and causes disharmony – such as stress – leads to illness, but that the imbalance can be treated by acupressure (p84), acupuncture, reflexology (p86) and/or herbalism (p136).

▶ Stand upright with your feet parallel and slightly more than hip-width apart. Raise your arms slowly above your head then trace a huge circle with your hands and arms by bending your body to the side and down to the floor, and up again.

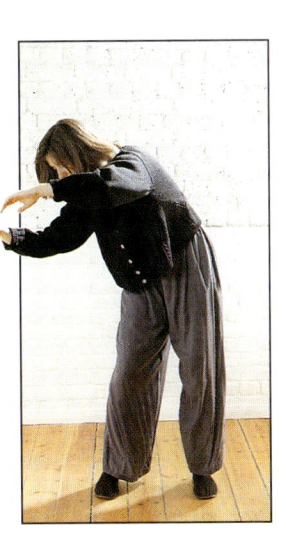

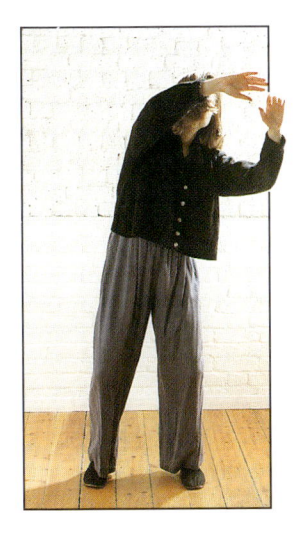

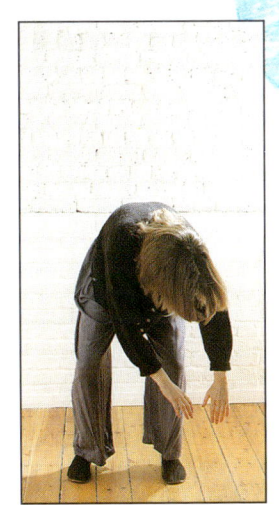

TECHNIQUES

THE ALEXANDER TECHNIQUE

Postural improvement, cure or prevention of a range of disorders, relaxation of mind and body and improved performance in various activities have all been claimed to result from learning the Alexander Technique. It was developed by F.M. Alexander, an Australian actor born in 1869, to overcome problems with his voice. As his career developed so did a recurrent problem with his voice which caused it to fail during performances.

Doctors were unable to help him and when he realized that the problem concerned the way that he used his voice, he decided to help himself. Using a mirror to observe his movements, Alexander's first discovery was that whenever he began to speak he pulled his head back and down. Over a long period of experimentation, he discovered that every performance of an act involves habitual patterns of movement of which we are normally unaware. To discover that you invoke a whole pattern of habitual and previously unobserved responses every time you wish to do anything comes as a surprise to most people who have not studied the Alexander Technique. Alexander would refer to the way that you carry out any act as your "pattern of use", so that you could have "poor use" or you could "maintain good use". He discovered that if he could "maintain good use" while speaking he experienced no more trouble with his voice.

He began teaching his technique for maintaining good use to other actors and singers. As he moved away from an acting career to a new career developing and teaching his technique, he began to see how wide its applications – and implications – were. Not only was good use necessary while speaking and singing, but all our movements – sitting, standing and walking – are affected by our habitual patterns of use.

Alexander taught his technique in Britain and America, gaining the support of actors, writers and philosophers. Of his four books, the third – *The Use of the Self* – is the most helpful. Much of his thinking, unconventional in his time, is now common currency and the technique has gradually gained the respect of many members of the medical profession.

In the hands of a skilful teacher, the nature of Alexander's technique can be glimpsed in a moment. The benefits of what is seen in that moment can be acquired progressively over a series of lessons. In the process of getting from "poor use" to "maintaining good use" your teacher will explain that old habits feel right – they are what has always felt right; old habits infect your whole use. So, the immediate resort to old patterns must be overcome. New patterns will feel strange and will make you aware of the relationship of the head, neck and back in all that you do. The technique is not just a way of sitting or standing up, nor is it simply a series of exercises. The teacher's hands and words together explain how to employ this technique of change. As you shed habitual patterns, your movements become freer, easier and more economical. A more complete sense of yourself leads to the disappearance of unnecessary muscular tension, much of which has locked you into bad postural habits. Headaches, neckaches and backaches which are the result of poor use will disappear. Breathing patterns will change. Frustration, anger, anxiety and worry and other habitual patterns of reaction, which are not always accurate and appropriate responses can be re-thought in the light of Alexander's teachings.

Common faults of posture
The ways in which you move are reflected in your posture. The model used on the following pages had no experience of Alexander Technique prior to the day on which all the pictures were taken. The pictures on this and the following page show common imbalances in most people's movements.

Standing

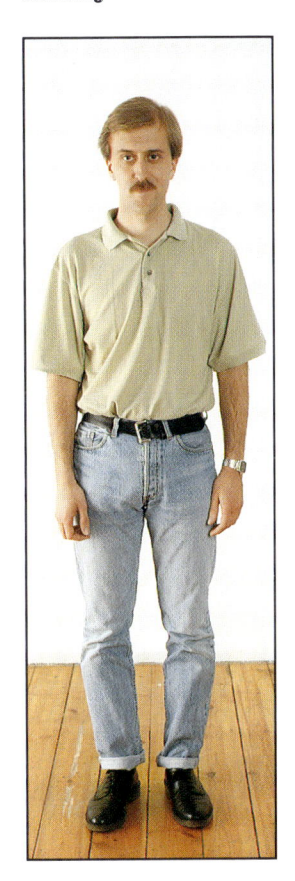

▲ Although this stance looks normal at first glance, it is unbalanced. The model's left arm hangs away from his body, his right arm hangs in, his right shoulder can be seen pushing forward, and you can see more at the right side than the left side of the neck.

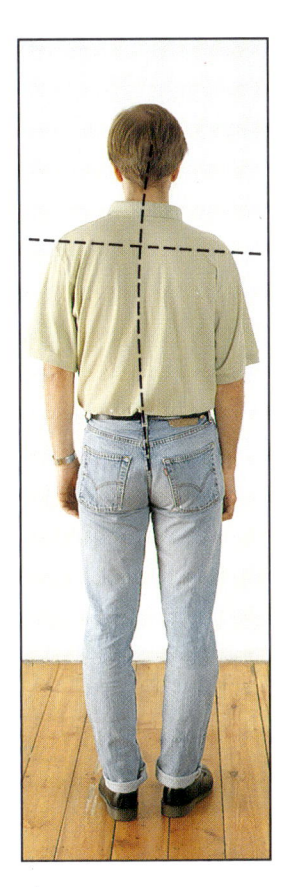

▲ The dotted lines show the curve of the spine, the head held off centre, and the raised left shoulder and the dropped right shoulder.

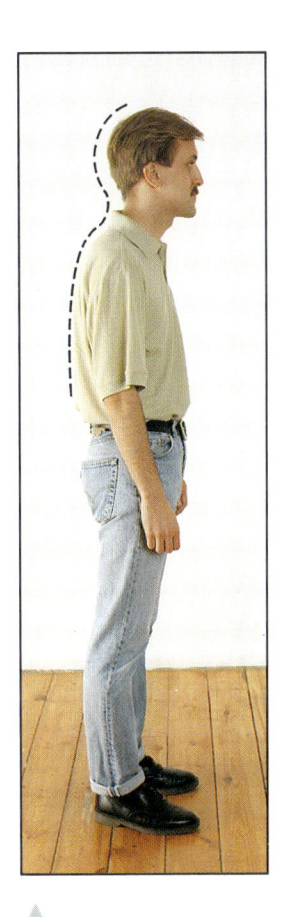

▲ The dotted line shows how the natural curves of the spine have become exaggerated, the neck curving forward, the upper back hunched.

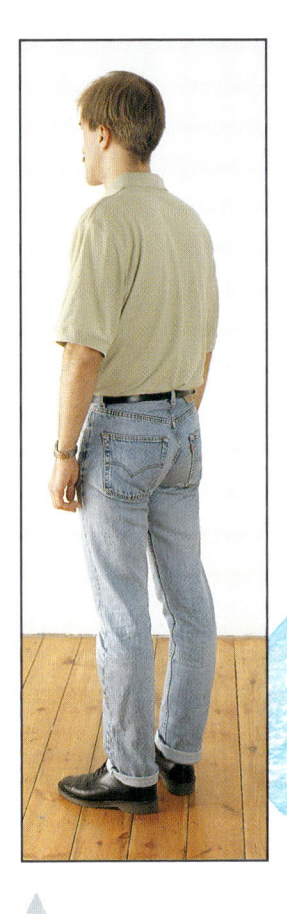

▲ The under curve of the upper back and the tension in the shoulders are visible again here. Another common habit is visible: the tendency to push the knees back so that the legs are braced.

WATCHPOINT

Begin studying with an accredited teacher. Teaching styles differ greatly but the underlying principle of Alexander Technique should become clear quickly.

TECHNIQUES

Sitting

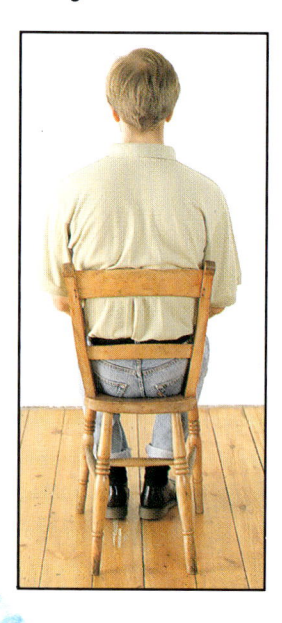

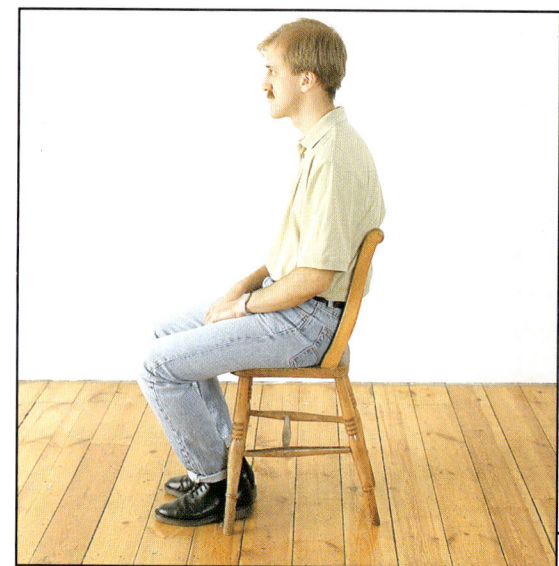

▶ Although these seated postures don't look too bad at first, if you look carefully you will see some of the same imbalances as on the previous page. Viewed from the side, the undue outward curve at the upper back and the exaggerated forward curve of the neck become clear. Notice how the model slumps into the back of the chair.

▶ Here the model was not expecting a picture to be taken – and settles even more into a habitual slump. The back is more rounded and, having allowed his knees to roll outwards, the model is resting on the outsides of his feet.

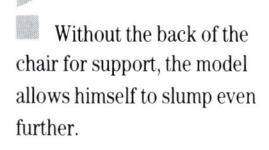

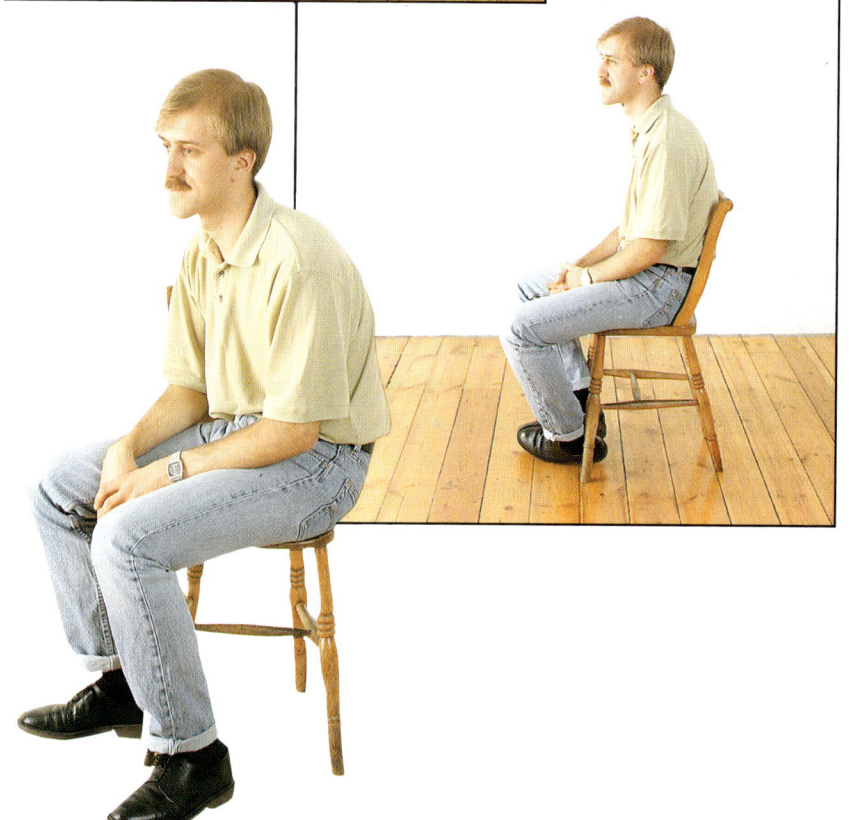

▶ Without the back of the chair for support, the model allows himself to slump even further.

104

ALEXANDER TECHNIQUE

Sitting down

These pictures show how the model goes about sitting down. Poor patterns of use are exhibited as the model sits down in his normal way.

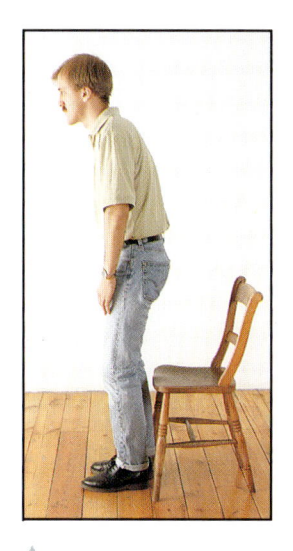

▲ This does not look too bad but the pattern of poor use is set.

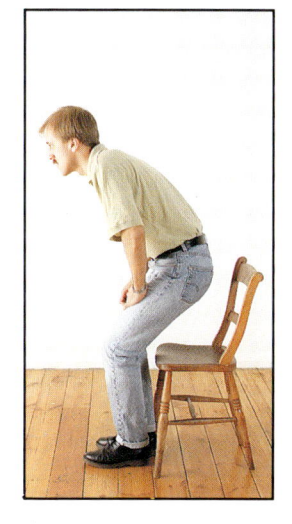

▲ The head is retracted and the back arched. Notice how the model puts hand on leg causing tension in the left shoulder.

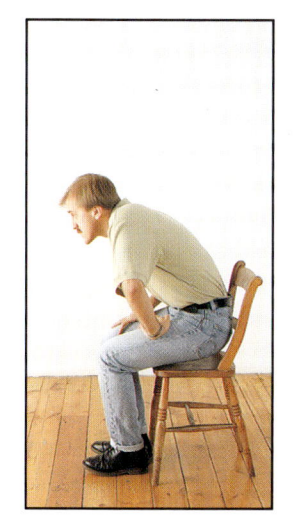

▲ He is nearly in a sitting position, with his head drawn right down into his shoulders.

After a short introductory session, the model allows the teacher to organize the act of sitting down. Afterwards the model agreed that he felt more comfortable and relaxed in the new seating position although to sustain this improvement would obviously take a number of lessons.

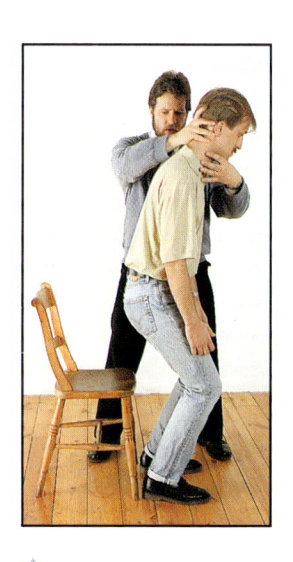

▲ Because the teacher is looking after the alignment of the head, neck and back, the head is no longer retracted and the back is less bent.

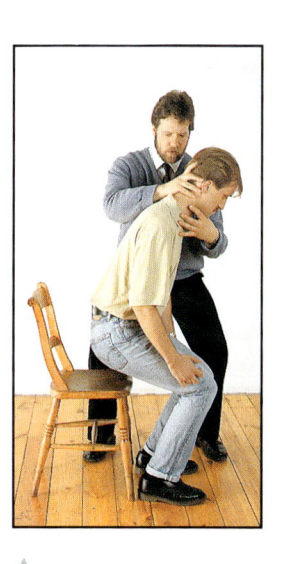

▲ As he sits, he stays more upright and keeps his head in line with his back.

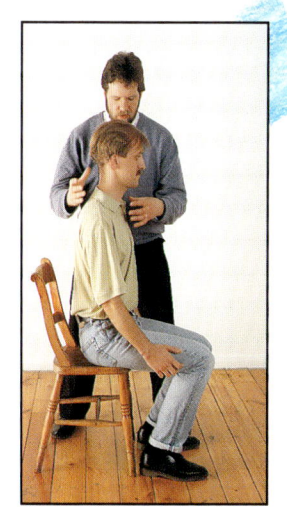

▲ He arrives in the chair sitting straight and in balance.

105

TECHNIQUES

Standing up
The model was asked to go about standing up in his usual way.

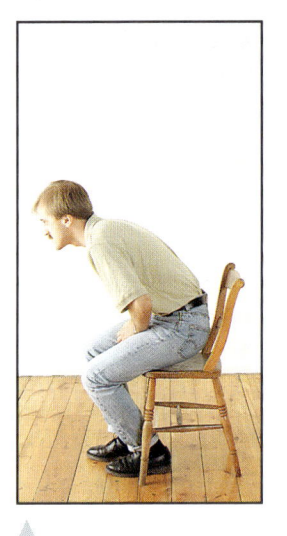

▲ The model leans forward, preparing to rise. To get off the chair he pulls his head back and hunches his back.

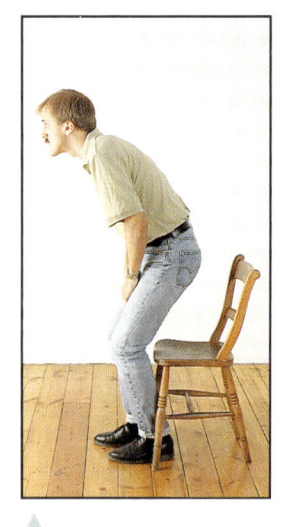

▲ This pattern is exaggerated as he rises.

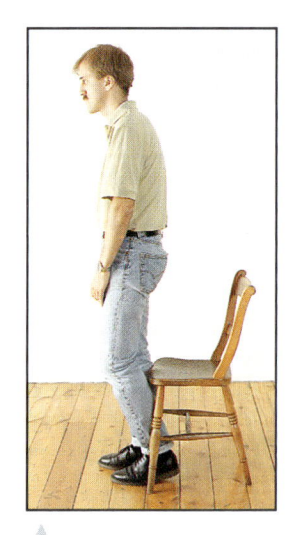

▲ This leads to his normal, poor standing posture.

Here the model allows the teacher to organize the act of standing, persuading the model not to respond in his old habitual way.

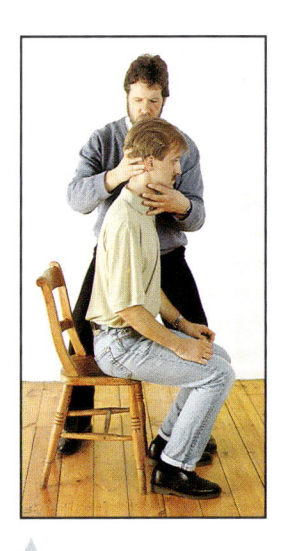

▲ The teacher prevents the model from pulling his head back.

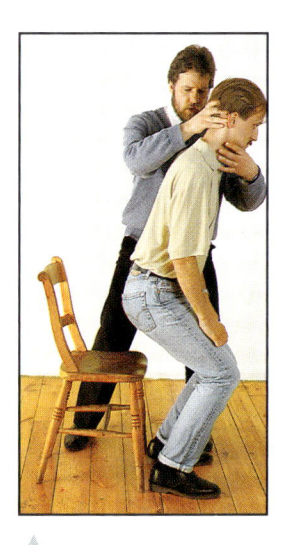

▲ Then he maintains the alignment of the head, neck and back while the model rises.

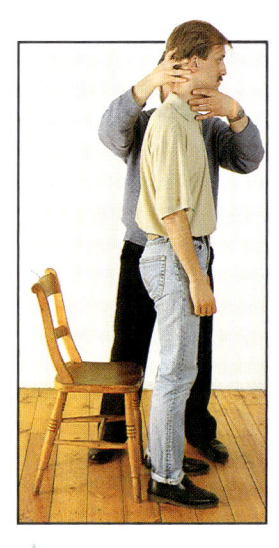

▲ The teacher helps the model to achieve a lengthened and more balanced standing posture.

106

ALEXANDER TECHNIQUE

Walking

Many characteristics of this model's manner of walking can be seen even in a sequence of still photographs, although they do not show how much his head moved backwards and forwards as he walked along.

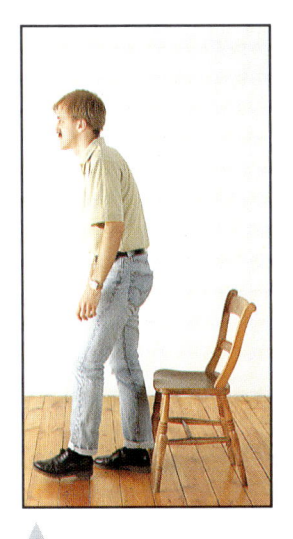

▲ To get started, he employs his usual pulling back of the head and hunching of the back. The whole movement has a downward tendency to it.

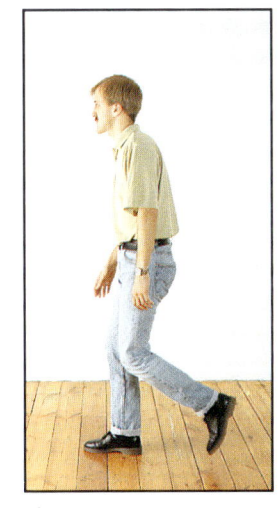

▲ In motion, the downward pull is still visible.

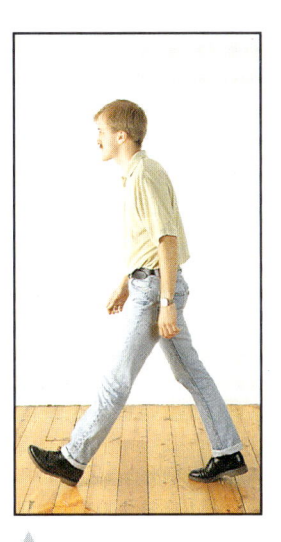

▲ Striding out, the chin pokes forwards, the chest points downwards. Notice the left leg thrown so far forward as to brace the knee.

The teacher pays attention to the relationship of the head, neck and back before attempting to demonstrate new patterns for walking.

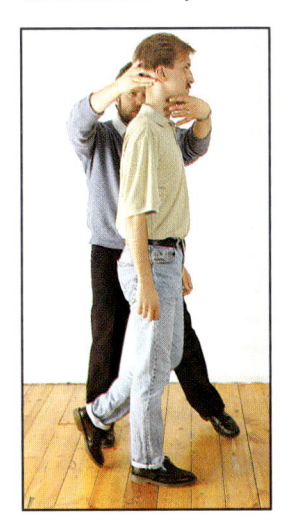

▲ The teacher leads the model into movement without the new pattern being lost.

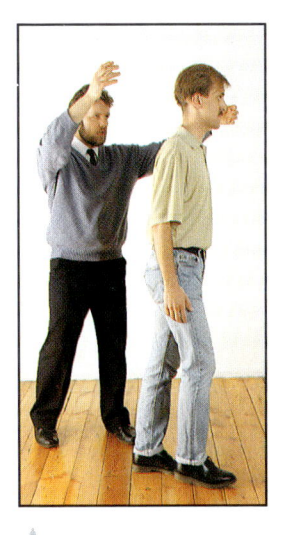

▲ As he continues with the movement, the model maintains some of his new-found poise.

107

TECHNIQUES

THE FELDENKRAIS METHOD

Moshe Feldenkrais, physicist (at the Sorbonne) and teacher of judo, escaped from Nazi-occupied France in 1940 and settled in Britain. After an injury cut short his sporting career, he started to study the dynamics of human movement, drawing on his knowledge of mechanics, anatomy and neurophysiology.

To some extent Feldenkrais combined elements of his scientific studies with his knowledge of the martial arts to develop a therapy based on the belief that movement and posture have a profound effect on mental and emotional conditions and are in turn affected by them. He believed that graceful movement could be re-discovered by stimulating the exploratory learning natural to infants and children.

Method

The Feldenkrais Technique can be learnt both in classes and in individual lessons. Pupils are encouraged to be aware of their bodies at all times and to sense the appropriate level of tension in their muscles – the aim is to produce natural, relaxed and easy movement. Students are taken through a sometimes complex series of movements, but some of the benefits that derive from them can be realized at home. The technique is suitable for people of any age.

WATCHPOINT

Pay attention to your breathing during each exercise – it should be even and uninterrupted. Concentrate on how each part of your body moves in relation to the others.

1. Start by lying on the floor on your back and sense how different parts of you make contact with the floor. Touch along the lower ribcage, noticing how an exaggerated curve in the lower back can push the ribs forward.

2. Bend your knees so that your feet are flat on the floor. Press with your feet slightly and lift your pelvis slowly away from the floor, feeling each vertebra come away from the floor until you reach the middle of your back and then slowly return to the floor vertebra by vertebra. Repeat this movement a few times gently, then rest, lying on your back again.

3. Bend your knees and slowly lift your pelvis again, vertebra by vertebra, until you reach the area of your upper back and shoulder blades and slowly let your pelvis return to the floor. Repeat a few times gently and slowly, then rest lying on your back.

4. With your knees bent and your feet flat to the floor, interlace your fingers and place your hands underneath your head. Bring your elbows toward one another and lift your head gently and slowly, feeling each of the vertebrae of the upper spine lift away from the floor and slowly return. Again, lie on your back and rest.

5. Bend your knees, interlace your fingers and place your hands underneath your head again and gently lift your pelvis once, then your head. Continue to alternate so that you "rock" up and down along your spine. Lie on your back and rest.

6. While lying on your back, touch with your hands along your lower back and notice that it lies more closely to the floor as the habitual muscular contractions in the lower back release.

7. Come slowly to standing and swing gently from side to side, noticing if this movement feels easier to you now and if your usual range of movement has increased.

FELDENKRAIS

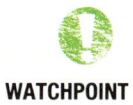

WATCHPOINT

The Feldenkrais Method is a gentle, gradual re-education of the way we move, but never a strain; movements should always be free and easy.

The gentle movements of the Feldenkrais Method are demonstrated as in stage 2 of the programme described on the previous page. Once you have been to some classes these exercises are suitable for practising at home.

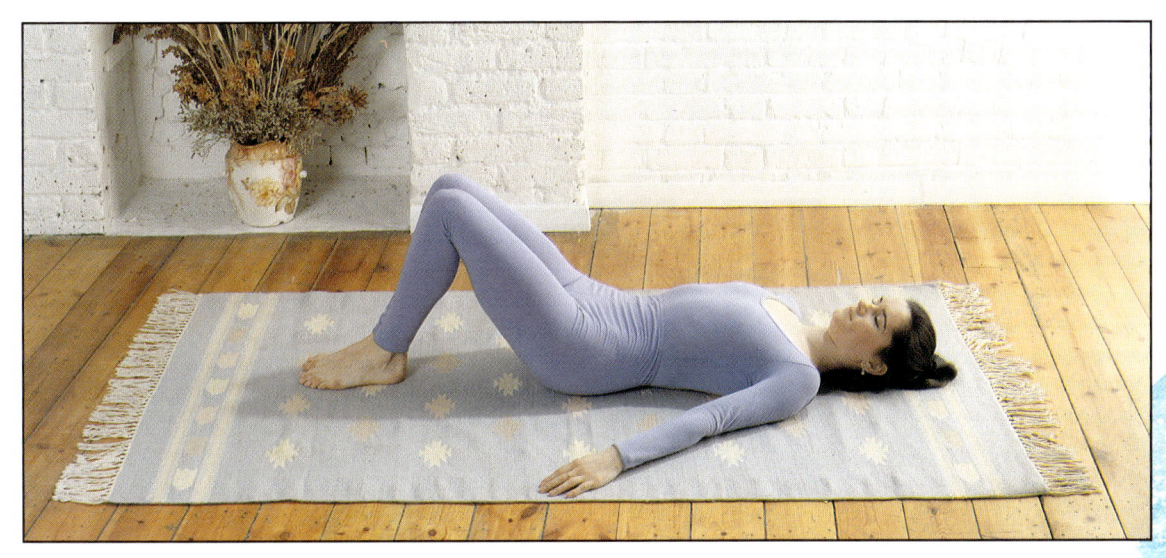

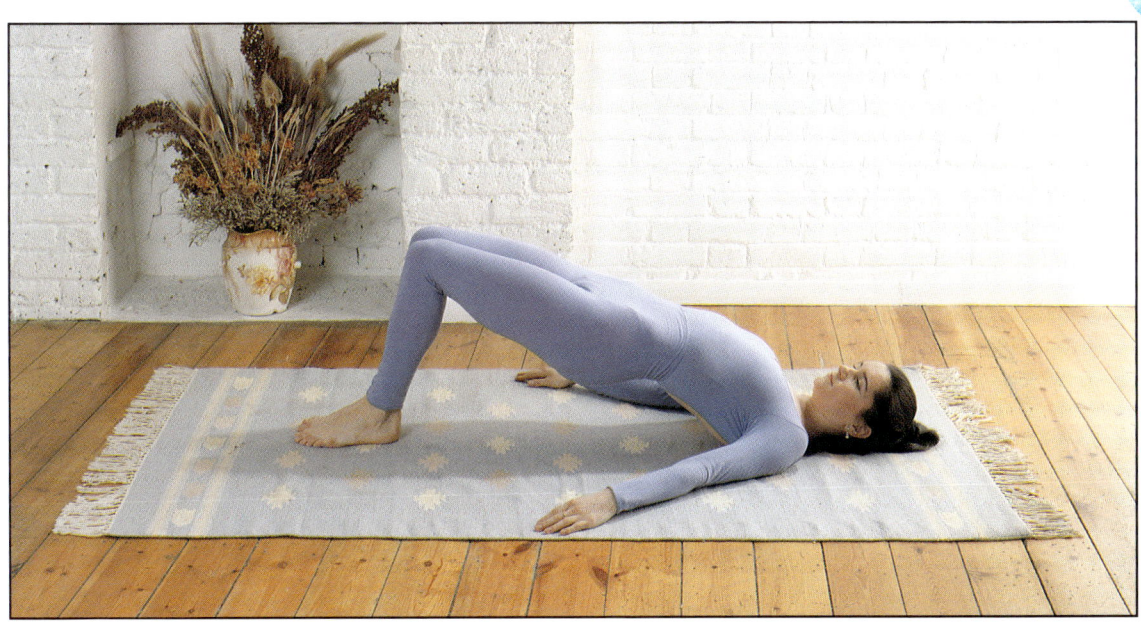

TECHNIQUES

YOGA

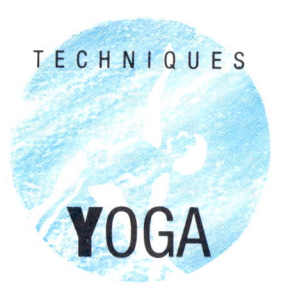

Yoga has been practised for thousands of years throughout the Indian sub-continent and is one of the six orthodox systems of Indian philosophy. The Indian sage Patanjali outlined the basic principles more than 2,000 years ago. According to him, there are eight stages (or limbs) in the quest for spiritual realization.

- Yama – universal moral principles including non-violence, truthfulness, chastity and absence of greed

- Niyama – purification of self through discipline and study

- Āsanas – the postures of Yoga

- Prānāyāma – the breathing techniques of Yoga

- Pratyāhāra – freeing the mind from the domination of the senses and of the distractions of the outside world

- Dhārana – deep concentration

- Dhyāna – meditation

- Samādhi – the state in which the soul is supreme

For a contented life you need a harmonious balance between your body, soul and mind, according to Yoga philosophy, and the pressures of modern society make it difficult to maintain an equilibrium. Many people who attend Yoga classes know little about the philosophy but still get great benefit from practising the postures (Āsanas) and breathing techniques (Prānāyāma). Yoga is particularly effective in combatting stress and stress-related illnesses as it helps both the body and the mind. By regular practice of the postures the body is strengthened and concentration is improved.

It is now commonly accepted by doctors in the West that Yoga can lower blood pressure, increase the body's strength and flexibility, and help to alleviate a wide range of problems including rheumatism and arthritis, back problems, menstrual disorders, migraine, and circulatory and digestive disorders.

There is no need to be young or physically fit to take up and benefit from Yoga. A qualified teacher will be able to advise you as to which postures will most help you and if any should be avoided – or if a doctor's advice is required before taking up Yoga.

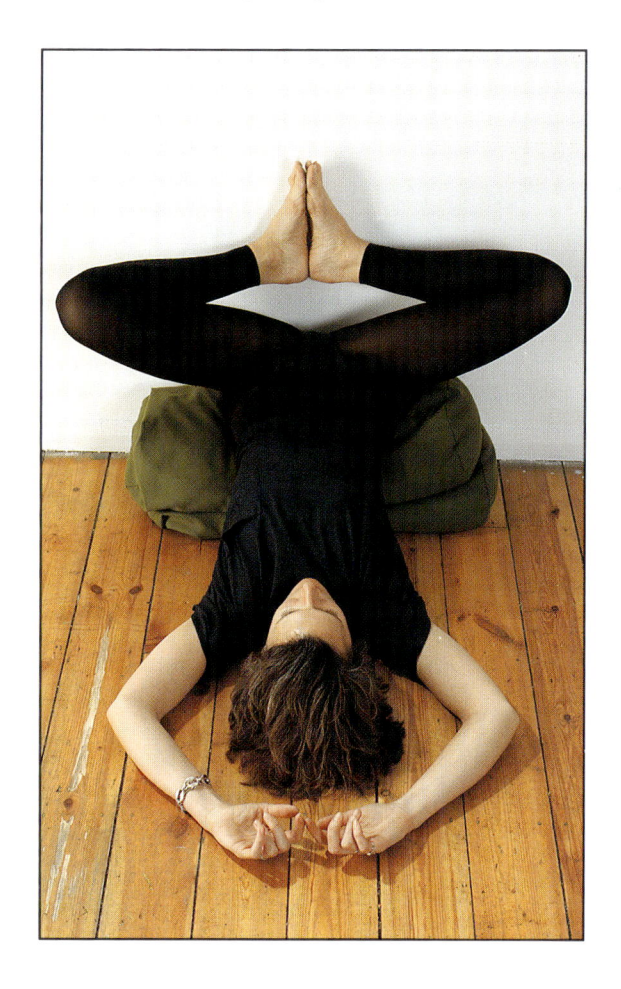

YOGA

WATCHPOINTS

If you have a medical condition check with your doctor before beginning Yoga classes. Begin studying with a qualified teacher. Don't practise after a heavy meal; wait for at least 3 to 4 hours. Don't do inverted poses during menstruation.

Yoga postures have their best effect if practised regularly – 15 minutes a day is adequate, but aim for half an hour or more, either first thing in the morning or in the evening. Different postures benefit different parts of the body and there are sequences of postures which are particularly suitable for relaxing, relieving dullness and depression, combatting insomnia, and so on. The three sequences given over the next six pages have been put together and executed by qualified yoga teachers.

Method

Provided you are learning with a qualified teacher, Yoga is a very suitable technique to practise at home. Ideally you need a quiet room and time free from interruptions, although Yoga does teach you to concentrate despite distractions. Wear loose, comfortable clothes and practise barefoot. Do not, though, practise on a slippery surface, as this can lead to accidents – if necessary use an exercise mat. Make sure that the room is warm, because warmth helps the relaxation and stretching of muscles.

Yoga poses are satisfying to do and attractive to look at. Don't despair if your first attempts are far from the poses pictured over the next few pages. Practice at any level is beneficial and flexibility improves surprisingly quickly if you practise.

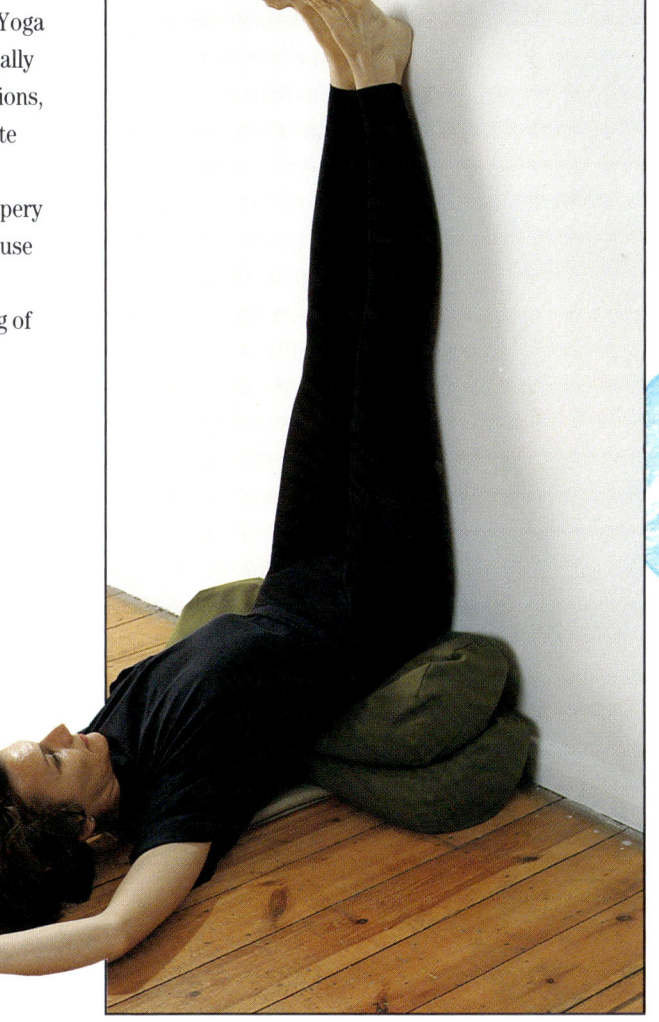

TECHNIQUES

Sequences

The following sequences of postures have been designed to relax you and also to relieve particular problems, like backache, mental fatigue or general tiredness. Each one ends with five minutes of relaxation. Always wear loose, comfortable clothing to practise, and make sure the surface is not slippery. If it is, use an exercise mat.

Remember if you have any medical condition, check with your doctor first before you practise these postures. The inverted poses must not be done during menstruation.

To refresh you

The sequence of postures on this page and the next will help you feel refreshed and are particularly good for tired legs.

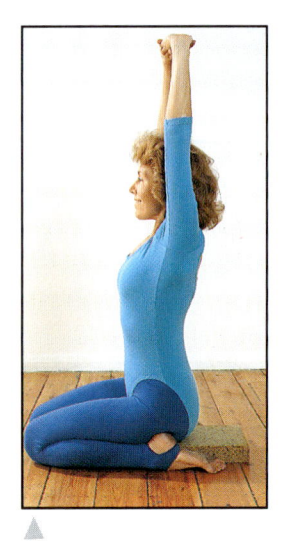

1 Parvatasana in Virasana: Sit on your heels. Pull your feet apart and sit on a folded blanket or support. Interlock your fingers (left over right) and stretch the arms forwards and upwards, palms outwards. Stay for 30 seconds and repeat with the fingers interlocked the other way.

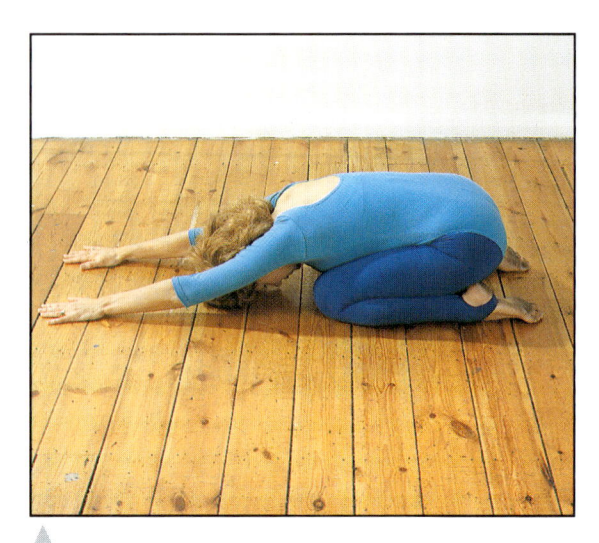

2 Virasana Forward Bend: After the previous posture, spread the knees apart. Extend the arms and trunk forwards until your forehead rests on the floor (if this is difficult, use a bolster). Stay for between 30 seconds and one minute.

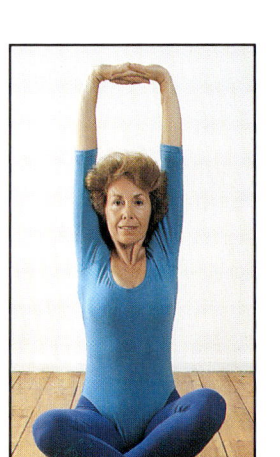

3 Parvatasana in Sukhasana: Sit upright with your legs simply crossed (right over left), your fingers interlocked (right over left) and your arms raised as in the previous posture. Stay for 30 seconds and repeat with legs and fingers crossed the other way.

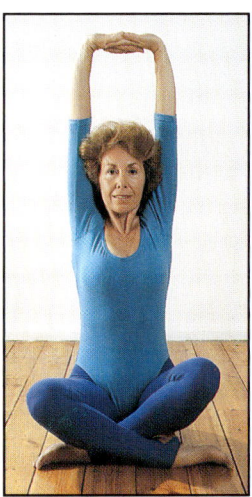

4 Sukhasana Forward Bend: Sit as for Sukhasana, left, and stretch the arms forwards on the floor until your forehead is touching it (if this is too difficult, use a bolster). Be careful not to strain your knees. Stay for 30 seconds and repeat with legs crossed the other way.

YOGA

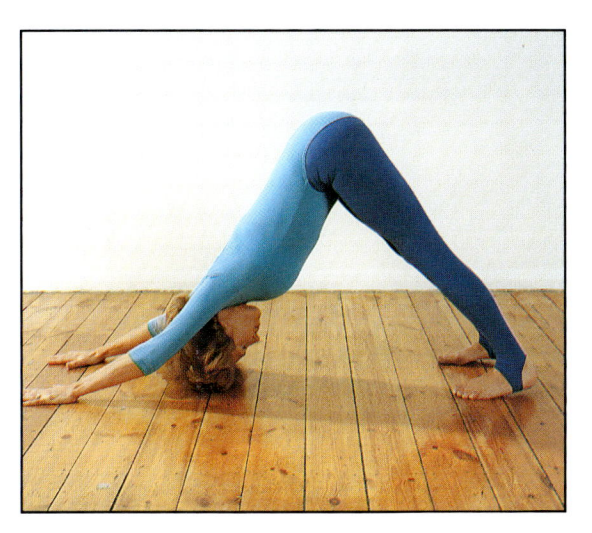

5. Adho Mukha Savasana: From a standing position, bend down and place your hands on the floor, a shoulder-width apart, and walk the feet back until the body froms an inverted 'V' shape. Keep the arms and legs straight and the hips lifted; the head should be relaxed. Stay for as long as you can maintain the stretch.

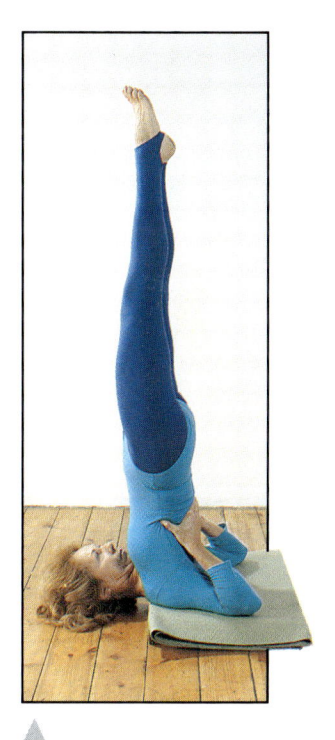

7. Ardha Halasana: From Sarvangasana, take your legs down onto a chair (with a folded blanket on the seat for padding and extra height). Take the arms over the head and relax completely. As in Sarvangasana, there should be no pressure or discomfort in your head, neck or throat. Stay for 5 minutes.

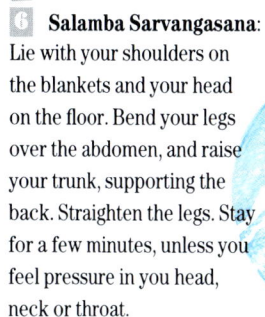

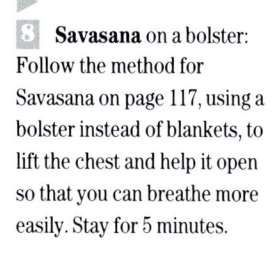

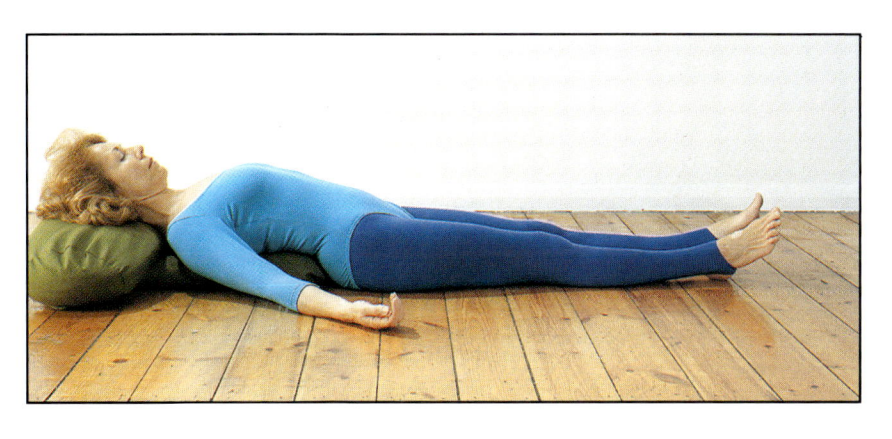

6. Salamba Sarvangasana: Lie with your shoulders on the blankets and your head on the floor. Bend your legs over the abdomen, and raise your trunk, supporting the back. Straighten the legs. Stay for a few minutes, unless you feel pressure in you head, neck or throat.

8. Savasana on a bolster: Follow the method for Savasana on page 117, using a bolster instead of blankets, to lift the chest and help it open so that you can breathe more easily. Stay for 5 minutes.

TECHNIQUES

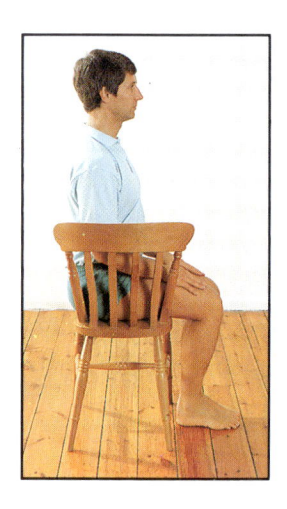

To relieve backache

1 Bharadvajasana (on chair): First sit sideways on a chair, your right hip towards the chair back, stretching the trunk up and with your shoulders back, and your legs and feet together.

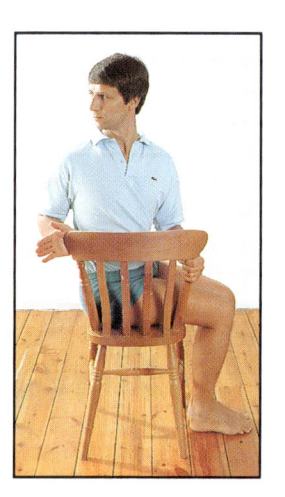

Then turn towards the back of the chair, placing both hands on the chair back, twisting your body to face the chair back by pulling with the left hand and pushing with the right. Stay for 30 seconds. Then repeat on the other side.

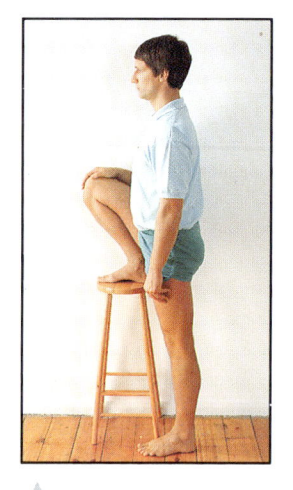

2 Maricysasana (standing): First stand in front of a stool, facing it, with your right side against the wall. Draw yourself up and place your right foot on the stool.

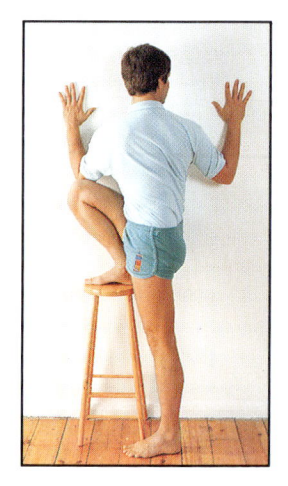

Then turn to the right and face the wall. Raise your arms and press your hands against the wall to turn the trunk to the right. Turn your head and look over your right shoulder. Stay for 30 seconds and repeat on the other side.

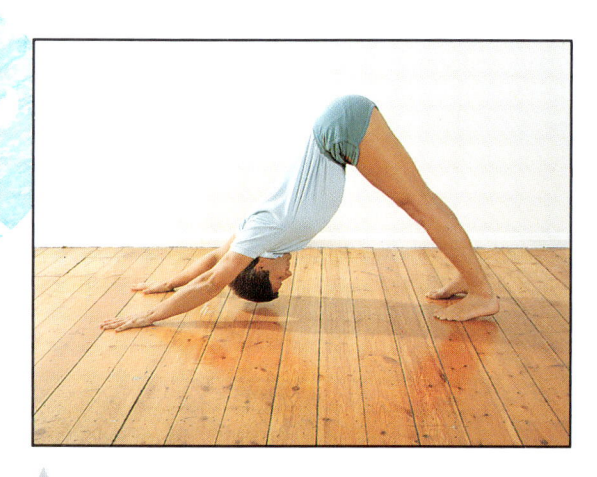

3 Adho Mukha Svanasana: From a standing position, bend down and place your hands on the floor, a shoulder-width apart, and walk the feet back until the body forms an inverted 'V' shape. Keep the arms and legs straight and the hips lifted; the head should be relaxed. Stay for as long as you can maintain the stretch.

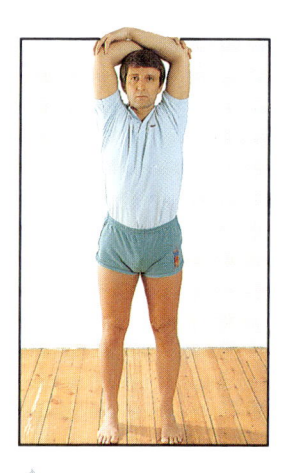

4 Uttanasana: First stand with your feet about 30cm (1ft) apart, clasping the elbows and stretching the arms up over the head.

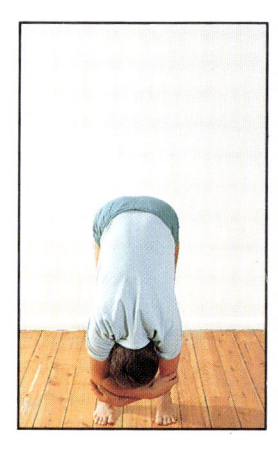

Then as you exhale, take the trunk and arms down while keeping your legs firmly stretched up and vertical. The head should be relaxed. Stay for 30 seconds.

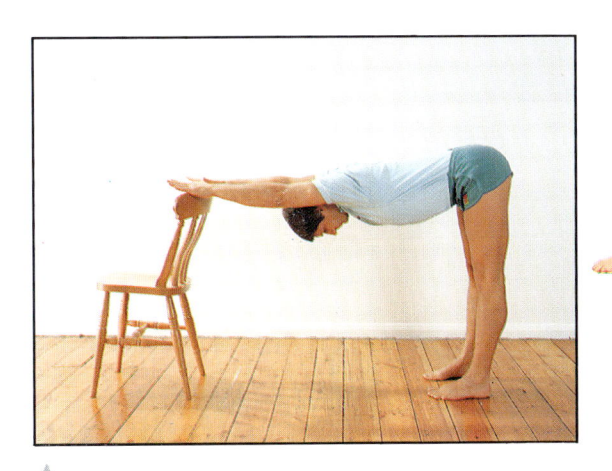

▲
5 **Uttanasana** (using a ledge): If you find it difficult to bend, then you can do Uttanasana with your hands on a ledge (or a chair back). Take the feet 30cm (1ft) apart. Stretch forwards and place the hands on a ledge at hip level. Keeping them perpendicular to the floor and straight. Stay for 30 seconds.

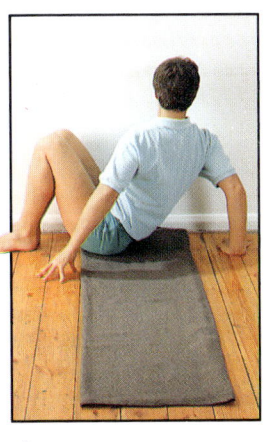

▲
6 **Urdhva Prasarita Padasana** (against a wall): First sit sideways on a mat with your hips as close as possible to the wall. Then lie down and straighten your legs, one by one, against the wall. You can take your arms up over head, palms upwards, or keep them beside the trunk. Stay for up to five minutes.

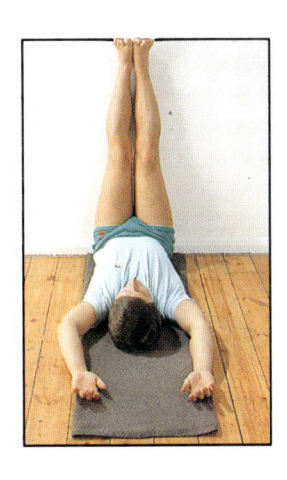

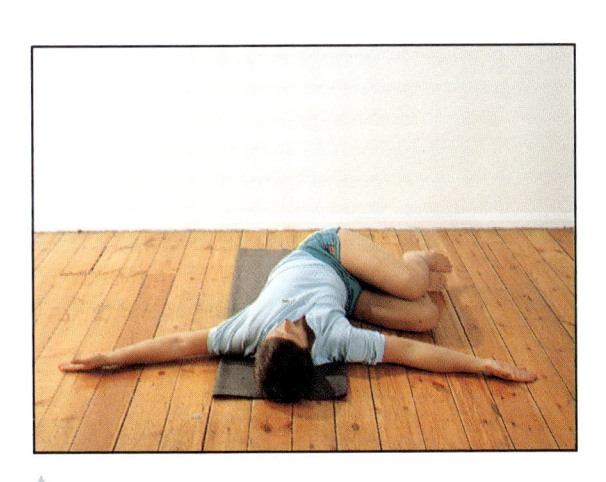

▲
7 **Jathara Parivartanasana** (with bent legs): Lie down on a mat, making sure you are straight. Stretch your arms out to the sides, palms uppermost. Bend the knees over the abdomen and take them down first to the right and then the left. Stay for 30 seconds each side.

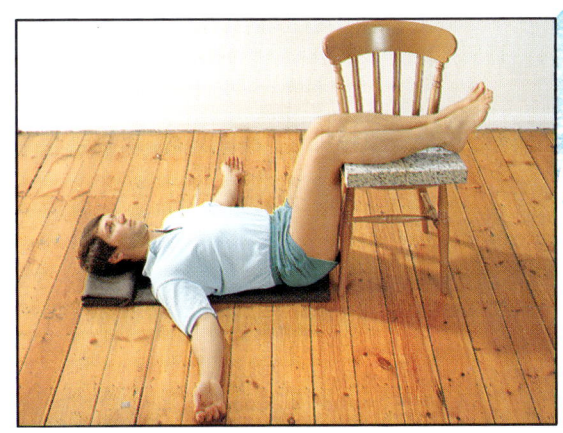

▲
8 **Savasana** (with your legs on a chair): Lie down on a mat near a chair. Bring your legs up and onto the seat, with the calves resting on the chair seat. (You may need to bring the chair nearer to you to make yourself comfortable). Stay for up to five minutes and turn to the side before getting up.

TECHNIQUES

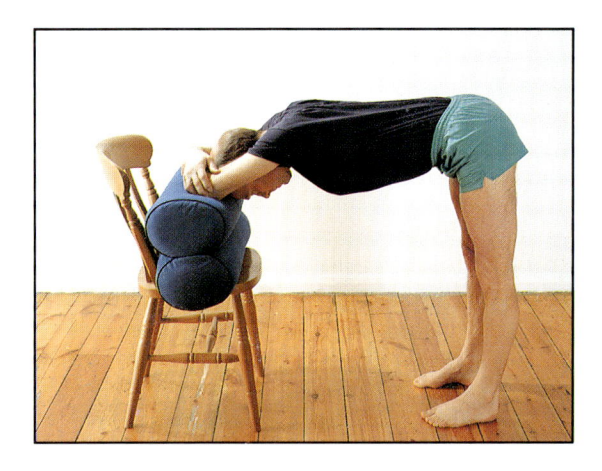

To relieve mental fatigue

1 Uttanasana (head supported): Stand with your feet about 30cm (1ft) apart, rest your head and arms on the chair. Enough cushions or a bolster should be placed on the seat so that you can stay comfortably in the posture for a minute or longer.

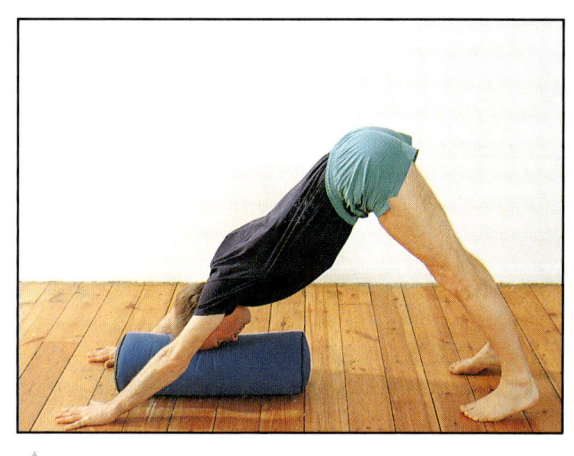

2 Adho Mukha Svanasana: Place a bolster on the floor, as shown. From a standing position, bend down and place your hands on the floor, a shoulder-width apart, and walk the feet back. Keep the arms and legs straight and the hips lifted; the head should be relaxed. Stay for as long as you can maintain the stretch.

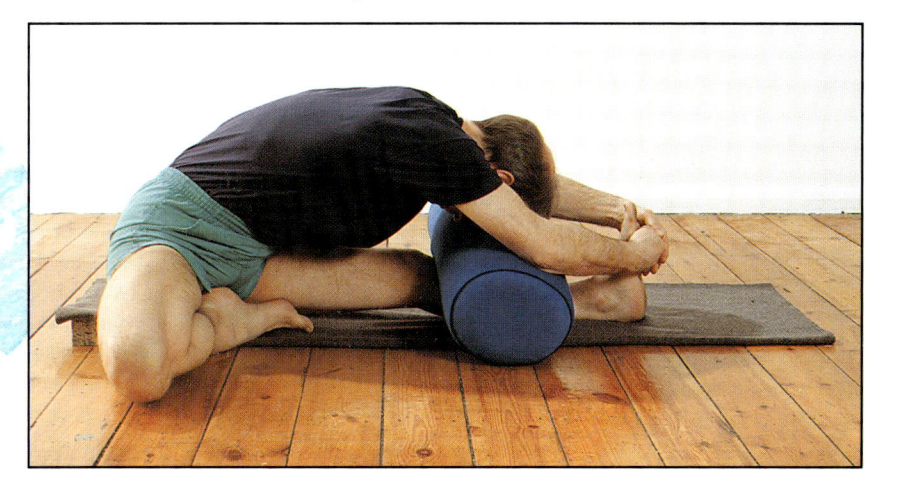

3 Janu Sirsasana: Sit erect, then bend your right knee with the heel against the groin. Place a bolster across your left shin and rest your head on it. Take your arms forward. You can either catch your foot with your hands (as shown) or rest your arms on the bolster. Stay for one minute or longer. Repeat stretching out the right leg and bending the left.

4 Triang Mukaikapada Pascimottansasa: Sit erect with your legs stretched out in front of you. Bend the right leg back, keeping the foot beside the thigh. Extend the left leg and place a bolster on the left knee. Stretch the arms, bend forward and rest your head on the bolster. As in the previous posture, you can either clasp the foot or rest your arms on the bolster. Stay for one minute or longer and repeat for the other side.

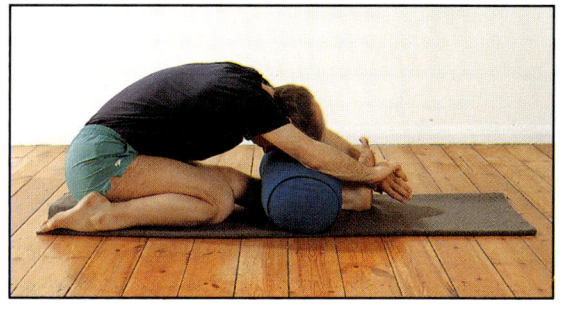

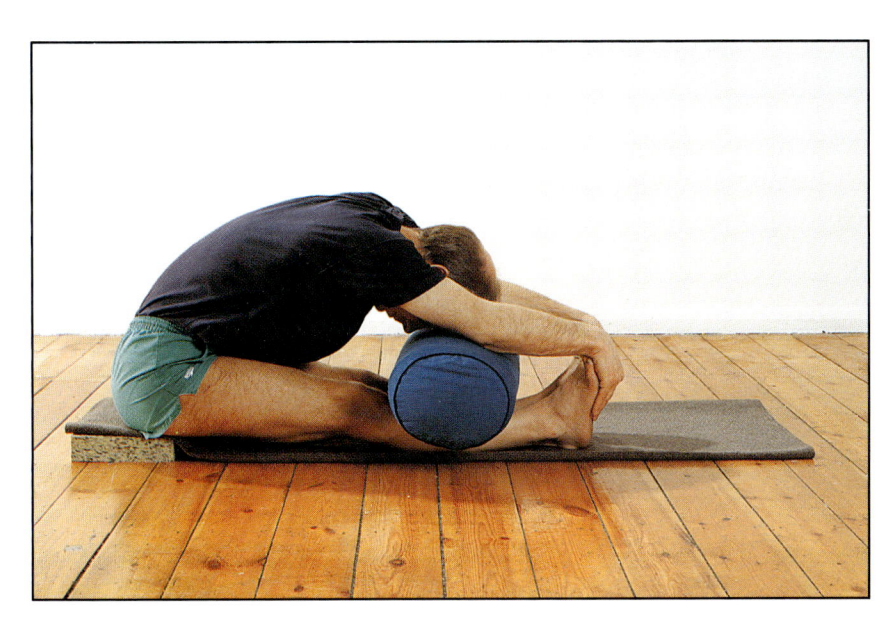

5 Pascimottanasana: Sit with your trunk erect and your legs together, stretched out in front of you. A bolster is placed across your shins. Bend forwards over the bolster until your forehead rests on it. (It is important for the forehead to rest, so if you cannot reach the bolster, use instead a low table with a blanket or cushion on it.) Stay for 30 seconds.

6 Setubandha Sarvangasana: Sit on the edge of a bolster and then lie back, keeping the bolster under the lower back. Take the arms over the head. If the back pinches, you can place a support under the feet to raise them to the same height as the bolster. Stay for a few minutes.

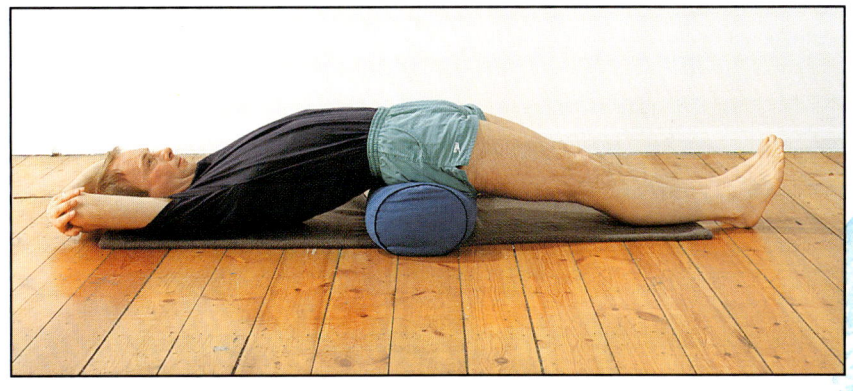

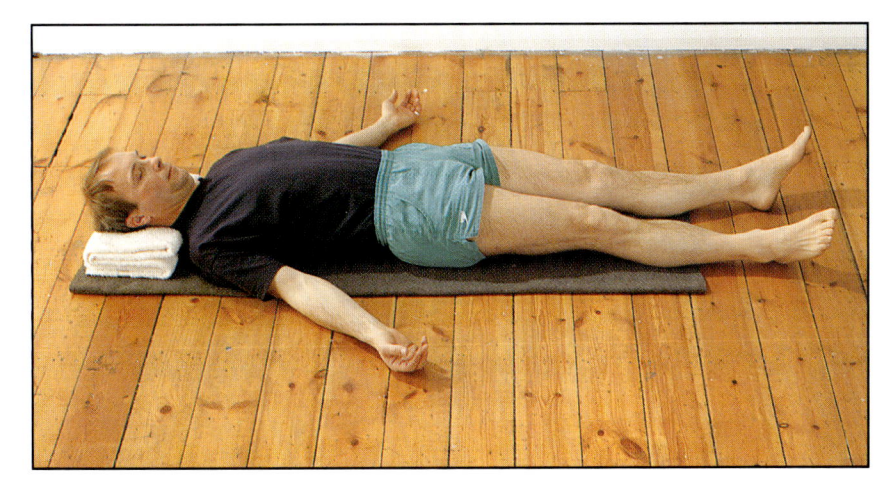

7 Savasana: Sit down with your legs stretched in front of you. Then lean back on your elbows, keeping your trunk and legs in line. Finally lie down with your head on the folded blanket, and extend your arms and legs prior to relaxing them. Turn your hands, palm upwards, and allow the legs to roll naturally out to the sides. Stay for five minutes or so.

TECHNIQUES

MEDITATION

Meditation is an ancient Eastern technique that has a similarity to self-hypnosis, in that it induces a trance-like state, which relaxes the mind and the body. Meditation became very popular – almost fashionable – in the West during the late 1960s and early 70s, being hailed as the answer to the stress of daily living. This enthusiasm was further fuelled when The Beatles started to follow the teachings of Maharishi Mahesh Yogi, a guru who taught a type of meditation he called transcendental meditation. As with many consciousness movements, though, meditation lost a certain degree of its popularity – in part because some forms have religious associations that many find hard to accept.

The theory is that every day your mind is filled with sights, sounds, smells and information; it has to evaluate all of these, to memorize some and act upon others. This enormous level of sensory input and the demands for analysis of it put a tremendous strain on the mind, which sometimes just cannot cope – the result being stress symptoms, and difficulty with relaxation. We are inclined to believe that sitting down in front of the television or reading a book is relaxing – it is physically relaxing, true, but the mind is still having to cope with new demands. Meditation cuts off the sensory input, halts the demands of the brain, and gives the mind a chance to rest. Research projects have shown that meditation can induce relaxation, lower blood pressure, reduce the body's metabolic rate and ameliorate many stress-related disorders.

So meditation is one method of relaxing the mind and triggering the body's own natural relaxation response – it is not necessary to follow the teachings of a guru or mystic to benefit from it.

Zazen (breath) meditation
This is a very simple technique and with practice you can use it anywhere – whether you are at work, on a journey or at home.

1 Choose your relaxation position and concentrate on your breathing, making it deep and even.

2 Next, empty your mind of everything but your breathing. Concentrate on the sensations of your ribs and stomach moving in and out (*see* Breathing).

3 To prevent your mind from wandering, you may find it useful to count up to ten as you breathe: inhale, exhale '*one*'; inhale, exhale '*two*'; and so on. Once you reach '*ten*', start at '*one*' once more.

4 As you count, fix your mind on one particular aspect of the breathing process – your stomach, for example, or your breastbone – to the exclusion of all else. This will help to deepen your level of relaxation.

5 If your mind begins to wander, just start concentrating and counting again. The more you practise the less often you will find that this is necessary.

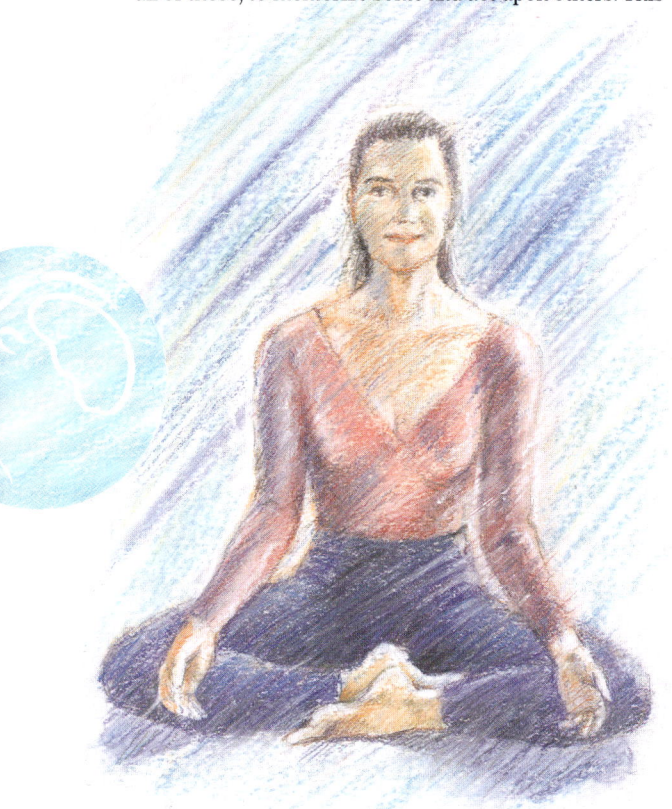

MEDITATION

Method
Before trying any of the techniques described below:

▪ make sure you will not be disturbed at all for at least 20 minutes;

▪ choose a relaxation position that suits you (*see* Basic Relaxation Techniques);

▪ relax and concentrate on your breathing.

Once you have learnt how to meditate, try applying your chosen technique twice a day, for five or ten minutes at a time, to keep stress at bay and increase relaxation. First thing in the morning, and straight after work or last thing at night are the ideal times, but the most important thing is to find your own ideal routine.

Mantra (word) meditation

Transcendental gurus believe that a mantra can only be given by a guru, but others believe that a mantra is just as effective if chosen by the individual concerned. Your mantra should be a word that has no relevance or meaning, a bland 'nothing' word. Dr Herbert Benson, an American from Harvard, suggested the word 'one' in his book *The Relaxation Response*; other good examples are *prana*, or *ch'i* (life force); and 'om' (the infinite, or 'God is love'). If one particular mantra does not appear to be effective after a few tries, choose a different word.

1 Relax in your chosen position, eyes closed.

2 Empty your mind and repeat your mantra as you breathe. Keep a steady rhythm.

3 Ignore all thoughts that enter your mind – if you cannot, and the rhythm of the mantra breaks down, just start again.

Trataka (object) meditation

The *trataka*, or object, is simply used as a device for focusing concentration, because so many people find it easiest to concentrate on a physical object outside and apart from themselves rather than on a word or part of the body. The technique described here is similar to that used in Visualization.

1 Choose a small object – it is traditional to choose a candle, partly because it is easy to concentrate on a light, which leaves an after-image in the eye; but any small object will do: a crystal, for example, or a shell, a stone or a ball.

2 Place your chosen object at a comfortable distance from the eye – normally a few feet away. The object should either be at eye-level or just below it, because the eye muscles quickly tire if they are forced to look upwards for any length of time.

3 Relax and breathe evenly and deeply. Look at the object and concentrate on it; feel its presence, focus on its shape, texture, weight and smell and sense its energy. Let these sensations float through your mind. Do not force them, though – the process is a completely passive one, involving 'seeing', not an intellectual exercise.

4 As for the other methods, if your mind wanders, just start to concentrate on the object again – with practise, this will happen less and less.

Bubble (thought) meditation

This is a slightly different form of meditation, because in it thoughts are allowed to enter the mind, having emptied it first.

1 As for the other methods, relax in your chosen position, breathe evenly and deeply and empty your mind.

2 Keep your mind empty for as long as possible, but when you have a thought, passively look at the thought, as though from the outside – without any judgement or emotion. Picture it in your mind's eye as surrounded by a bubble.

3 As you look at the bubble, let it drift slowly up into the sky until it disappears from sight, over about 30 seconds.

4 Empty your mind again. Wait until the next thought comes and then repeat the same procedure.

5 At first you will find that your mind is a jumble of thoughts and impressions, but they will gradually dissolve, and you will be able to keep an open mind for long periods.

6 One bonus of this technique is that solutions to difficult, worrying problems often enter your mind unaided.

TECHNIQUES

AUTOSUGGESTION/COUÉISM

Emile Coué (1857–1926), a French chemist and psychotherapist, suggested that it was not hypnotism that achieved cures, but the patient's own imagination stimulated by the hypnotism. The theory grew out of his analysis of a newly patented medicine that had completely cured one of his patients, which proved to be little more than coloured water. Coué began to investigate and work with the idea of recuperative autosuggestion – that if you sow a positive or health-giving thought in your subconscious mind, the body's own recuperative powers will be reinforced and do the rest. The concept is similar to that of autogenic therapy.

Emile Coué's practice is best remembered through the 'mantra' he popularized – 'every day in every way I am getting better and better'. Serving as a significant part of the method, the phrase encapsulates the theory: that all of us have wellsprings of healing energy which can be tapped through a current of words – interpreted according to need – that suggest cure. Serving as the incantation to the imagination, the reinforcing phrase seeps through to the subconscious mind where the healing forces can be rallied.

Autosuggestion has been found to be highly effective in the treatment of many stress-related problems, both physical and mental, especially in cases of anxiety, obsessive behaviour, drinking, smoking, over-eating and a weakened ability to cope with life in general.

Method

1 Relax the whole body and clear the mind of worries using one of the techniques below.
- Basic Relaxation Technique
- Autogenic Therapy
- Meditation

2 List the factors relating to your life that you wish to modify, making sure that your motivation is not in conflict with your conscious desires, then list the reasons why you then wish to change these factors.

3 Write down simple phrases that sum up the changes required. Ensure that they are all positive, since any negative phrase will only accentuate the problem. *'I will not eat too much'*, for example, is not the correct phrase, since it will reinforce the idea that you do eat too much. Say instead *'I like small portions'*. This idea is similar to the one that underpins the concept of positive affirmations, as used in self-hypnosis.

4 If you feel stressed or 'down', and wherever you are and whenever it is, repeat Emile Coué's phrase – or make up a specific one of your own.

5 Write down a list of positive phrases and keep them in your pocket – read them, or merely feel the paper to remind you of them, whenever you feel tension or the need to reaffirm the changes in lifestyle and attitude that you are trying to attain gradually.

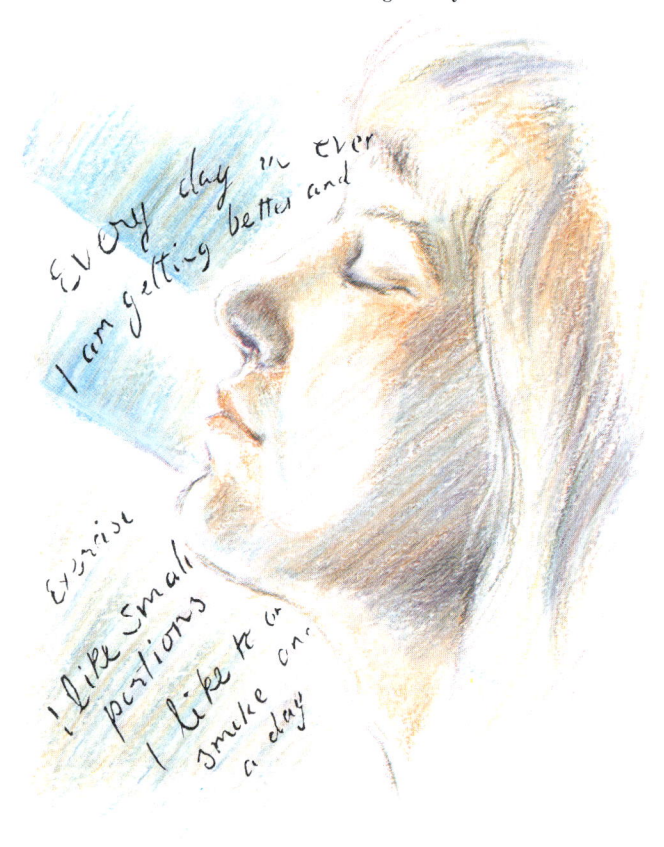

Autogenic Therapy

Johannes Schults, a German psychiatrist working in the 1930s, discovered that some of his patients could put themselves into a light hypnotic trance and that when they did so these patients responded better and more quickly to treatment – even when no positive suggestion or command had been given by a therapist concerning a specific problem.

Schults devised a system of relaxation that he called autogenic therapy, in which he recommended six specific commands that the patient would repeat slowly in sequence; the system is still in use today. When the patient has achieved the desired effect for each command, he or she moves on to the next command. Once all six commands have been given and the effects achieved, the patient relaxes into a semi-hypnotic state. Schults believed that once the body was in the relaxed state its in-built powers of self-healing would automatically tackle any problems. Successive practitioners have refined the technique by allying it to the use of positive affirmations (see Autosuggestion), once the patient has learnt how to reach a light hypnotic trance at will (*see* Self-Hypnosis and Visualization).

Autogenic therapy is usually practised by licensed practitioners, but with commitment the technique can be employed at home – it is most useful in the treatment of stress-related symptoms and is very effective in inducing relaxation.

Method

1. Lie down and relax as in the Basic Relaxation Technique.

2. Relax, breathe deeply and slowly, and repeat the following six commands under your breath; repeat each command until the desired result is felt and then continue to the next one.
   "*My legs and arms are heavy.*"
   "*My legs and arms are warm.*"
   "*My heart is steady and calm.*"
   "*My breathing is regular and calm.*"
   "*My abdomen is relaxed and warm.*"
   "*My forehead is cool and clear.*"
   It may take quite a few sessions to achieve the correct state of relaxation, but it is worth persevering, since this is such a simple technique that can be practised anywhere – sitting at work, for example – and it will leave you feeling calm and capable.

3. Once you are completely relaxed repeat the command that has the closest bearing on your problem.
   "*My forehead is cool and clear*", for headaches.
   "*My stomach or abdomen is relaxed and warm*", for digestive problems.
   Otherwise, make up your own commands, to fit your personal problems;
   "*My mind is clear and strong*", for example, for lack of concentration.
   "*My whole body is relaxed and warm*", for insomnia.

4. As you repeat your positive command, cross your fingers – this will emphasize the command and with practice you can simply repeat the command in your head and cross your fingers to bring relief, for example, from a headache, sudden tension or anger. This quick relief is useful when at work, travelling or during a hectic time at home, and will only take five minutes or less.

5. To begin with, aim to set aside 30 minutes three times a week to practise the technique. Once you can relax deeply and fully, practice as and when required – though try to put aside half an hour once a week.

TECHNIQUES

VISUALIZATION THERAPY

In general terms, visualization therapy is a technique by which the body's own healing mechanisms are stimulated by conjuring up in the mind visual images of positive and pleasant objects or scenes.

It has long been accepted that the subconscious mind, which controls the body's internal mechanisms, can be influenced by imagination and suggestion. Witch doctors and voodoo priests, for example, have used this link for centuries, both to maintain discipline and to heal – if a witch doctor tells someone that he or she will die, that person may well die if the belief in the witch doctor is strong enough. By the same token, people who are told that they have been given cures may well, in fact, achieve cures if they truly believe in the power of the person administering them. The principle works in Western societies, too – placebos (inactive tablets) often work when they are prescribed by conventional doctors.

Visualization is a simple technique that is purely an extension of what we all do throughout our lives: day-dreaming of what has been and what we wish to happen. The difference is that visualization is more focused and intense. In both complementary and conventional medicine today, the technique is used as part of the strategy against a number of diseases, and against cancer in particular: sufferers are asked to picture the body's own disease-fighting cells as knights on white chargers, for example, and to focus on the image of these knights attacking and defeating invading cancerous cells.

For our purposes, though, visualization need not be as intense as this. Instead of dreaming about the might-have-been or the might-be, you use your day-dreams to help you combat stressful situations, improve your self-image and to realize your potential. You can use the technique too, to defuse a potentially stressful situation by rehearsing different relaxing scenarios in the imagination. In fact, though visualization can help in all conditions, mental or physical, it is particularly effective in combating stress.

Method

First, relax, having made sure that you will remain undisturbed, in a position that is comfortable for you (*see* Basic Relaxation Technique).

For general relaxation

1. Close your eyes and imagine a beautiful, calm scene – perhaps a place you have visited, a painting that particularly appeals or a pleasant and relaxing social situation. Imagine all the details in the scene: feel the temperature, see the colours, hear the sounds, smell the fragrances.

2. When your mind wanders, bring it firmly back to your scene. Concentrate on the image and make every effort to exclude everything else – this may be difficult at first, but becomes easier with practice.

3. Try repeating some positive affirmations, previously rehearsed, to yourself (*see* Autosuggestion *or* Self-hypnosis). Make sure the affirmations do not disrupt the scene, but help to endorse the feeling of peace and relaxation. For example:-
"*I feel warm and relaxed.*"
"*I am content with myself.*"
"*This scene makes me feel good.*"
"*I feel at peace.*"
"*I am mentally and physically relaxed.*"

For stress at work

If you know that you have a stressful meeting or a confrontation coming up at work, prepare yourself in advance.

1. Relax at home a few days beforehand, and visualize the meeting – the room, the people present and the agenda.

2. Rehearse the various scenarios in your mind, trying to cover every eventuality. Picture what it is that will produce the stress, however small and petty these details seem to be – elements may turn out to be important in a way you had not realized.

VISUALIZATION

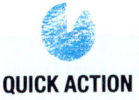

QUICK ACTION

Keep a photograph of your chosen scene, or of something similar in your bag or your pocket. When you start to feel tense, take the picture out – imagine yourself in the scene, blank out everything else, relax and let the tension ebb away. If you practise this at home you will find that it only takes five minutes, wherever you are.

3 Distance yourself from the problem and relax, breathing deeply and evenly. At first, you will find that tension rises, but if you persevere you will feel it draining away.

4 Once you have confronted and overcome one problem, go on to the next.

By the time the meeting takes place, you will have defused the situation in your own mind, and you will feel little or no stress.

The technique of imagining an obnoxious boss or a difficult colleague in a situation that is embarrassing or even humiliating for him or her is a tried and tested one, and is, in fact, part of visualization. Imagine your boss in the bath, or think of your difficult colleague in an uncomfortable meeting with the tax authorities – you will find that this helps reduce both the stress that they trigger in you and any feelings of inferiority that they may inspire.

For stress in social situations

Use the same techniques as given above for stress at work to reduce the stresses you may encounter in social situations and to combat shyness or a feeling of inferiority. Repeat positive affirmations to yourself as you imagine the occasion (*see* Self-hypnosis *and* Autosuggestion).

"*I am confident.*"
"*I am relaxed.*"
"*I am enjoying myself.*"
"*I am friendly.*"
"*The people I meet are friendly.*"

For stress at home

At home, relax and visualize yourself coping cheerfully and well in spite of all the demands placed on you. Visualize your house when it is organized and clean, repairs have been made, the shopping has been done, you are getting on well with the people you live with, the children are happy, and so on. If one situation, in particular, produces tension, rehearse it in your mind as above, until you can think of it without any rise in tension.

To relieve a particular symptom, either mental or physical

Visualize yourself as being well, fit and healthy. If you have a stomach-ache, for example, never think of yourself in terms of suffering from a stomach-ache and unable to work or enjoy yourself, but concentrate on a positive image of yourself as healthy, pain-free and capable of doing anything.

If you take a pill, for a headache for example, visualize its ingredients as soldiers in a powerful army, ready and waiting to fight the pain in your head. Visualize the army as it attacks and defeats the pain, rapidly and efficiently.

Visualize your body as strong and healthy, and your mind as clear and powerful. Characterize your body's own healing powers as invincible, capable of maintaining your health and helping you to combat any stress, so that you feel calm and relaxed.

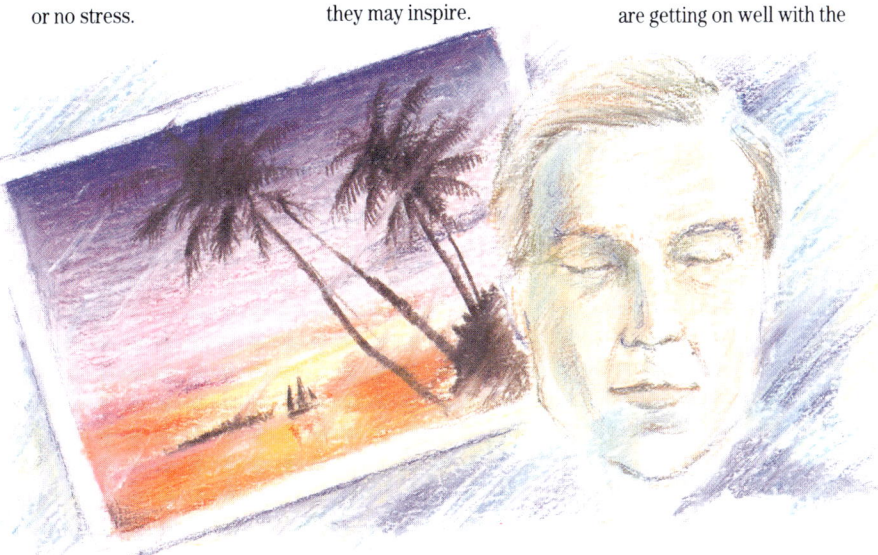

TECHNIQUES

SELF-HEALING

The ability of one person to heal another by the 'laying on of hands' or through thought transference has been recognized and practised in cultures throughout the world. Unfortunately, healing has also been connected in many people's minds with occultism and even witchcraft. Since the third century AD the Christian Church has always been very sceptical of 'miracle' cures.

Recently there has been a tremendous resurgence of interest in healing, as people have been disillusioned with orthodox medicine. Britain has always been a centre for healers, because the British medical profession, though disapproving in many cases of the practice, has always felt that it is unnecessary to legislate against a treatment that cannot cause any harm – some doctors even refer patients to healers. On the Continent there is tremendous interest in healing, but the practice is against the law in most countries, though often tacitly tolerated. In America only medical practitioners and pastors are allowed to lay on hands, though healing is not itself illegal and the Federation of American Spiritual Healers is a well-known organization.

There are two types of healing, though there is often an overlap between them: first, faith healing, in which the patient puts complete trust and faith in the healer and allows the healer's own healing energy to flow into his or her body; second, spiritual healing, in which the healer acts as a medium, transmitting the innate energy of the universe – the life force that is perceived and named in a variety of ways across different cultures and religions – to the patient. Spiritual healing does not require any spiritual faith on the part of the patient; in fact, it can be performed without the patient's knowledge.

Method

1. Relax in one of the basic relaxation positions.

2. Place your hands in the prayer position, a few inches apart.

3. Concentrate on your hands and on the space between them. You may well feel what is almost a pull between your hands.

4. Keep concentrating on this for a few minutes, then place your hands on your head – the bottom of the palms of the hands just touching the top of the ear lobes.

5. Feel the touch of your hands on your head. Sense the energy flowing through your head from one hand to another.

6. Stay like this for a few minutes – or until your arms ache.

7. Remove your hands and assume the prayer position again; hold this for a few minutes.

8. Place your hands on any part of your body that hurts or is troubled. Your stomach, for instance, if you suffer from irritable bowel syndrome, diarrhoea or constipation. Move your hands to your head in the case of a headache, or place your hands on your chest to relieve anxiety and tension.

9. Let your hands rest lightly and firmly on the chosen part of the body for about five minutes. Concentrate on your hands and feel the warm energy flow between them and around them.

10. After five minutes, relax quietly for a short while.

Many scientific papers have been written in an attempt to analyze reports of 'miraculous' cures performed by healers. Most people now believe that there are certain people that can, by some method as yet not understood, give a form of curative energy to all living things – animals as well as people. One healer, whose work was reported in the scientific press, was shown to have kept red blood cells alive long after they should have died when placed in a saline solution; there are many other instances of similar occurrences. Some people believe that the methodology involves 'energy imprinting': positive thought transference that passes from the healer to increase the patient's own 'energy' level, enabling a 'self-cure'. Whatever it is that happens, it is correct to say that many healers feel completely exhausted after healing – especially in the case of faith healing, in which the practitioner passes his or her own energy to the patient.

One possible reason for the success of faith healing is that many diseases are psychosomatic – in other words, the symptoms are real but the cause is in the mind – and that the course of a disease is always affected by the attitude of the patient to the disease and to life itself. As a result, most symptoms of a disease (and this is particularly true of stress-related disorders) will be helped by the feeling that one is cared for and cherished: a loving touch can be just as effective in some conditions as the techniques of conventional medicine.

It is not strictly necessary to visit a healer, however. Everyone has the potential to become a healer, and so to heal themselves. All mothers know, for example, that a kiss on a child's hurt will 'cure'; a cuddle will soothe upsets and solve problems. You, too, can experiment with the healing properties of touch, applied in the correct way, to help relieve stress and promote relaxation.

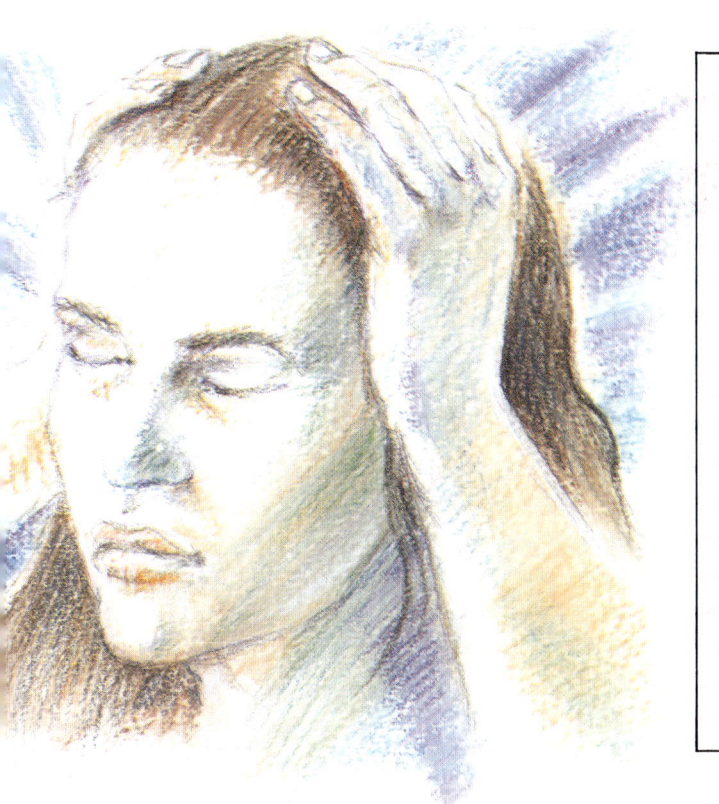

Guidelines

▪ All the above techniques can be very effective when performed by a willing partner who believes in what he or she is doing.

▪ If you have a spiritual faith, think about the life-giving spiritual force that is strengthening your own energy as you lay on hands.

▪ Some people feel a glowing warmth, a tingling or a sensation of 'knots' relaxing; not everybody feels this, though, so do not worry if you do not.

▪ Many people feel the benefit of healing very quickly; others need to repeat the technique twice weekly for a few weeks before it has any effect.

TECHNIQUES

SELF-HYPNOSIS/HYPNOTHERAPY

Self-hypnosis is a form of therapy that uses hypnosis as a tool in dealing with disorders of an emotional content. It is most effective in relieving stress disorders – high blood-pressure, migraine, insomnia and asthma in particular – and help break addictive habits.

When hypnotized, a subject is in a trance-like state in which the mind readily accepts ideas, resulting in a focusing of attention and a reduction of the ability to make conscious decisions; this state is one of total mental concentration, yet complete physical relaxation. Many therapists agree that simple techniques of auto-hypnosis (as outlined here) can be used to benefit many cases of psychsomatic illness.

The true father of modern hypnotism was an Austrian called Franz Anton Mesmer (1734–1815). Mesmer believed that an unseen power affected human behaviour – he thought it came from the planets – and that this power could be harnessed by one person to control the mind of another; he named this effect mesmerism. Mesmer's ideas gained almost immediate public acceptance. Mesmer's ideas of an outside power were, of course, nonsense, but his treatment was sometimes effective, since he implanted the idea of a cure in his patients' minds.

Partly as a result of Mesmer's ideas, there is still a degree of suspicion about hypnotism that lingers; the art has also suffered from its inclusion in music hall acts, and its portrayal in literature – the character Svengali, for example, in Georges du Maurier's *Trilby*, of 1894. Gradually, though, hypnotism came to be accepted by conventional medicine in the treatment of certain psychosomatic and mental disorders, and in the last few decades it has become one of the most popular of the complementary medical techniques. Today, the art is taught in reputable colleges in most countries, and it is used in the treatment of a wide range of disorders.

It is important to remember that hypnotism is not really a treatment in itself, but is an induced state in which the mind readily accepts the ideas that are suggested to it; on 'awakening' – though the subject is fully conscious throughout – the ideas are incorporated. A light hypnotic state, however, involving just 30 minutes of your time, can result in a feeling of calmness, relaxation and mental agility – similar to the feeling you have after a really good night's sleep.

But how does hypnotism work? For simplicity, let us accept that the brain is divided into two parts: the conscious mind and the subconscious mind. The conscious part controls and evaluates the world outside and sends messages and commands to the subconscious. The subconscious mind is similar to a computer; it has no critical faculty and accepts everything that is told by the conscious mind as a fact – even if it is not a fact; once an idea is implanted in the subconscious mind, though, the conscious mind has extreme difficulty in overriding it. For example, people who were bitten by dogs when young may have had implanted in their subconscious minds the thought that dogs are dangerous; they will believe this implicitly, even though the conscious mind logically tells them that the majority of dogs are friendly.

This relationship is significant, since the subconscious mind also regulates the involuntary systems in our body: circulation, for example, breathing and our emotions. When the conscious mind has implanted ideas in the subconscious mind that lead to

WATCHPOINT

Self-hypnosis should only be practiced on the advice of a therapist. Read this complete section before trying to start hypnosis.

QUICK ACTION

When you feel stressed, whether at work, at home or in a social situation, relax, shut your eyes for a moment, breathe deeply and evenly and repeat your phrase or word to yourself a few times. Then open your eyes and continue with what you were doing.

stress and tension, it is sometimes very difficult to shift them – even when using the various techniques of physical and mental relaxation. This is one reason why, for example, we find it difficult to change set habits, such as smoking and nail-biting, even when we really want to.

Self-hypnotism is a way of safely by-passing the conscious mind and reaching the subconscious mind. In self-hypnosis you are not trying to delve into your subconscious, but to plant positive thoughts, desires and ideas into it. With perseverance, the subconscious mind will accept these as fact, and make both the conscious mind and the involuntary systems behave accordingly. This means that self-hypnotism is an excellent way of combating stress-related symptoms and of increasing the body's ability to relax and cope, mentally and physically.

Method

Before attempting to achieve a light hypnotic trance, you must relax physically and try to convince yourself that

WATCHPOINT

You can buy tapes that help with self-hypnosis, but make sure they are recorded by a reputable, trained hypnotherapist.

Guidelines For Success

1 To maximize the chance of success, any new ideas introduced to the subconscious should be:

- genuine – it is no good asking your own subconscious to do anything that you honestly do not want to do;
- simple and positive – for example you should say to yourself *"I am confident"* not *"I will not be nervous"*, *"I am relaxed at work"*, not *"I will not be tense at work"*;
- use the present tense – even if it sounds odd;
- make sure that the idea refers to an action not an ability – for example *"I will sleep well and deeply"*, not *"I can (or am able to) sleep well"*;
- only try to implant one or two new ideas at any one time.

2 Write down the suggestion you wish to implant on a piece of paper, following the guidelines above. When they are clear and accurate, either record them on tape, or, after reading and visualizing them in your mind's eye, think of a short phrase that sums up what you have written. For example: *"Sleep soundly"*; *"I am relaxed and happy"*; *"I concentrate well"*; *"I am friendly and sociable"*; *"I am well"*; and so on. Use this word or phrase to implant the idea in your subconscious.

3 Make your own tape. Record a basic relaxation technique that works for you, follow it with the self-hypnotic technique described above; include the affirmations used at each session and then your personal affirmations; finish by recording the commands that bring you out of the trance.

you can hypnotize yourself. Remember that it is impossible to be hypnotized unless you consciously want this to happen. Try not to be sceptical, frightened or over-analytical about the process. Once you have learnt how to hypnotize yourself, practice will enable you to put yourself in a 'trance' whenever you wish to, quickly and easily. Try the Basic Relaxation Technique, meditation or autosuggestion to relax for self-hypnosis.

1. Once you are feeling relaxed and comfortable, select a small stationary object – one that forces the eyes to look up just slightly. Fix your attention on the object and empty your mind to everything else. Then repeat commands to yourself:
- **Command:** *"My eyelids are becoming heavier and heavier – they will gradually close."* Once they have closed, concentrate on your breathing – it should be deep and even.
- **Command:** *"I will relax more deeply every time I breathe out."* Deepen the trance by slower and deeper breathing.

2. Visualize an up-and-down movement: a swing, for example, a see-saw or the pendulum of a clock; follow its swing in your mind's eye.

3. Count down, slowly and in a dull monotone, from ten to one, saying *"sleep now"* after each number: *"ten, sleep now; nine, sleep now"* and so on. At *"one"* you will be in a light hypnotic trance – completely conscious, but relaxed. Your conscious mind will be in neutral, unwilling to make the effort to do anything.

4. At this point, repeat the following affirmations to yourself – they do not have to be word perfect as long as you can visualize them:
- **Affirmation:** *"In any emergency, I will come out of the trance quickly and easily and be able to cope with the situation immediately."*
- **Affirmation:** *"I will stay in this hypnotic trance for"* – set your own time limit for this, though not longer than 30 minutes – *"and then I will bring myself out of the trance."*
- **Affirmation:** *"I will stay in a light or medium trance and not sink to a deep trance."*
- **Affirmation:** *"I will not fall into a trance in a situation in which it might be dangerous to do so"* – while driving, for example.
- **Affirmation:** *"I will find it easier and easier to relax and hypnotize myself."*

5. After you have repeated these affirmations, continue with your own personal affirmations, then allow yourself to relax completely before you bring yourself out of hypnosis.

6. To come out of self-hypnosis, simply count up, in an increasingly positive way, from one to five; between each number say *"When I wake I will feel relaxed, calm and full of life."* At "five" you will be completely awake. Enjoy how you feel, before moving.

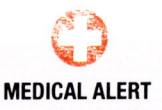

MEDICAL ALERT

Psychotic and severely mentally unstable people should never attempt self-hypnosis.
Never implant a possibly dangerous idea. If you say, *"I will drive"*, for example, it is possible that you will try to drive before you have learnt how to.
If you visit a hypnotist, ensure that he or she is well-qualified and registered with the appropriate national body.

Other Trance Triggers

There are a number of routines you can use to put yourself in a trance. Try them all and see which one is right for you – or devise one.

- First, follow the basic technique for relaxation.
- Imagine that you are descending from the top of tall building in a lift, and that you are watching each number light up in turn. Feel the lift slowing down as you near the bottom. Tell yourself that you will be hypnotized by the time you reach the ground.
- Imagine you are climbing down a spiral staircase. With each step you will relax more deeply and by the bottom you will be in a light hypnotic trance.

Biofeedback

In essence, biofeedback is a scientific technique that serves to prove to the more sceptical Western mind that Eastern healers who suggested that the human mind could influence, and, to a certain extent, control the autonomic nervous system of the body – the involuntary system that regulates heartbeat, blood circulation and the action of the digestive system – might well have been on the right track all along.

Biofeedback was formulated during the 1960s, when special machines were invented that could monitor a person's heartbeat (the electrocardiograph, or ECG), brain waves (the electroencephalograph, or EEG) and general levels of relaxation, and display these on a visual display unit (VDU). Before long, it had been demonstrated that a subject could alter blood pressure, brain wave patterns and level of relaxation by watching the VDU and 'willing' the desired response. Some people have shown the ability to go further than this: by controlling the amount of acid produced in the stomach, for example, to prevent or cure ulcers.

Research has shown that once someone has seen for themselves that they can relax or lower their blood pressure with the aid of biofeedback equipment, that person will be enabled to influence his or her own autonomic processes to achieve the same results without the use of the machinery.

Method

You can try biofeedback training at specialist centres – these can be found in many large cities, especially in the US, and an increasing number have been established in Europe over recent years.

A number of commercial biofeedback machines are available for use at home. The simplest, and the most successful when it comes to treating stress, is called a relaxometer. This is relatively cheap, small (the size of a transistor radio) and easy to use. Two small electrodes are attached to the palm of the hand, the machine is turned on to produce a tone or click that is then relayed through earphones to indicate your level of relaxation. The tone is something of a whine when stress levels are high; but given concentration, will and determination you should, with practice, be able to lower the pitch to a pleasant buzz, indicating a successful reduction in stress levels.

Once you have proved to your own satisfaction that you can reduce stress as shown by the relaxometer, try to achieve the same results without its use.

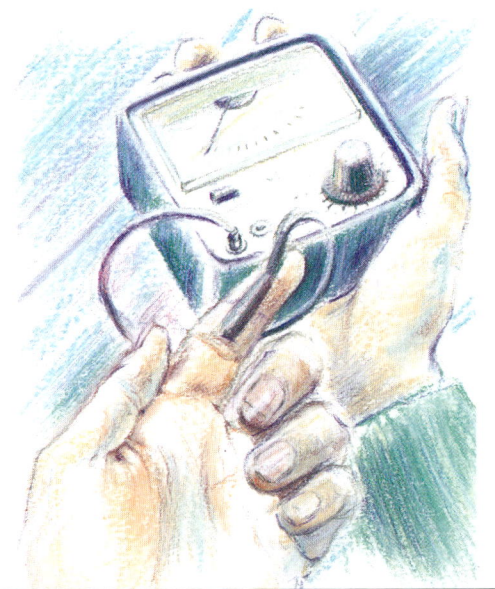

TECHNIQUES

NUTRITIONAL MEDICINE

A form of therapy also known as clinical ecology, in which the diet is adapted in order to improve both physical and mental health. Each individual has different nutritional requirements, and, of course, the requirement changes according to age, sex, activity and stress levels. But all of us need to take various vitamins, minerals, fats, proteins, carbohydrates, fibre and water regularly in order to maintain the body. When a person is under stress, the body needs an increased amount of particular nutrients, and an inadequate intake will exacerbate the signs and symptoms of stress.

It is now generally recognized that in the Western world we eat too much highly refined food, that is grown with the help of toxic chemical fertilizers and pesticides and contains artificial additives and colourings. The standard Western diet also includes too much animal fat, processed foods, sugar, salt, refined flour, tea, coffee and alcohol, and lacks sufficient fibre.

This sounds rather daunting. But you do not have to eat a boring, restrictive diet to make sure that the body receives all the nutrients it requires. Simple food in its natural, unrefined state is health-giving and delicious too! A gradual change in eating habits is more effective than a drastic overnight change, which is rarely maintained. In order to begin improving your diet choose from the guidelines for improved eating below, and gradually alter your habits in line with the recommendations. For example, if you drink too much caffeine, begin reducing your intake to below 5 cups a day by replacing every second cup with herbal tea or other non-caffeine alternatives. A good way to kick off an improved eating regimen is to go through your cupboards and throw out any foods that are high in sugars, fats, and salt.

Recommendations

1. Eat a varied, interesting diet – include some of your favourite foods.

2. Eat as much fresh food as possible – do not overcook vegetables or fruit. Steam rather than boil in order to reduce the loss of vitamins through cooking.

3. Avoid highly refined foods and foods containing additives and food dyes especially orange and yellow colourings.

4. Cut down on your intake of red meat; trim any fat off meat and grill, bake, or sauté, rather than fry.

5. Cut your intake of refined sugar and carbohydrates down to a minimum – that means sweets, chocolate, cakes, biscuits, jam, soft drinks and ice-cream should be replaced with sugar-free, wholemeal alternatives.

6. Reduce the quantity of fats in your diet, both those that are visible and those that are not – 'hidden fats' are found in dairy products, processed meat, pies and sausages.

7. Make sure that there is sufficient fibre in your diet. Fibre is found in fresh fruit, wholemeal bread, pulses, beans, wholegrain cereals and fresh or lightly cooked vegetables.

8. Reduce your consumption of animal protein replacing it with the proteins found in fish, poultry, nuts, beans, peas and other vegetables. These proteins are also rich in essential vitamins and minerals.

9. Limit your intake of stimulants such as coffee, tea and alcohol. Five cups of drinks containing caffeine (colas too) should be the daily maximum; 2 to 3 cups would be better. Limit alcoholic drinks to 3 to 6 per week as a maximum.

10. Stop smoking. Among other things, smoking inhibits the absorption of minerals and vitamins.

Nutrition For Stress

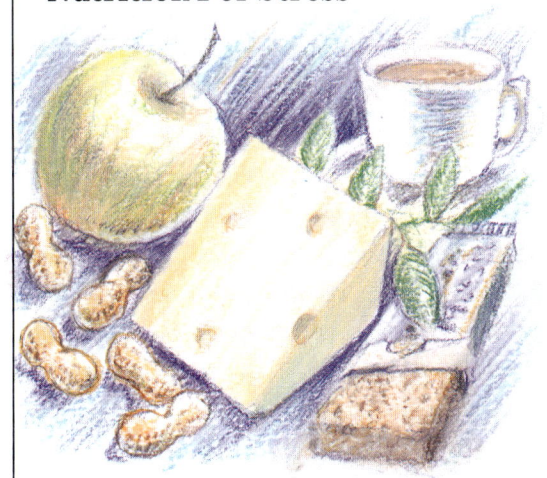

1. Eat regular meals to prevent your blood sugar level from falling – this can cause palpitations, panic attacks, anxiety, insomnia, headaches and emotional swings and instability, and is often the result of eating too much refined carbohydrate. Three meals a day that contain the right balance of essential nutrients is still the best regime, along with healthy snacks to boost blood sugar levels. Characteristically, blood sugar dips at mid-morning and mid-afternoon, so eat peanuts, an apple, cheese or a sugar-free muesli bar at these times.

2. Avoid junk food in the form of high sugar, salted snacks such as crisps, candy bars and ice lollipops.

3. Cut caffeine out of your diet – it is found in tea, coffee, dark chocolate and cola. This is especially important in the evening if you suffer from insomnia, anxiety and mood swings. Buy caffeine-free alternatives. Caffeine reduces the absorption of iron from vegetables, if drunk at meal times, and can cause or increase all the symptoms of stress. Until the body has adapted to the withdrawal of caffeine it is common to feel tired and have headaches, but these should pass within three days. Some herbal teas are very good for relaxation, such as camomile and sweet marjoram for headaches.

4. Limit your intake of alcohol, or cut it out altogether. Alcohol often helps people to relax temporarily but only increases the symptoms of stress in the long run. It is absorbed by the body in the form of refined carbohydrate and damages the absorption of many vitamins, especially those of the B group, and some minerals, such as zinc, magnesium and calcium. A moderate amount of alcohol – 3 to 6 drinks a week should be your maximum.

5. Do not eat a large meal late at night just before going to bed.

6. Take dietary supplements when you are under stress in order to ensure an adequate intake of nutrients. These can be bought at most chemists and health food shops. The supplements to use are: vitamin B complex; vitamin C; calcium; magnesium and zinc. Avoid vitamin B just before bedtime, as it can be a stimulant.

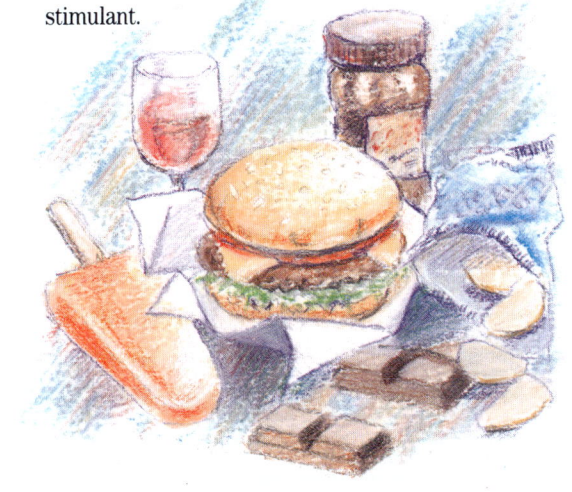

High-Nutrient Foods

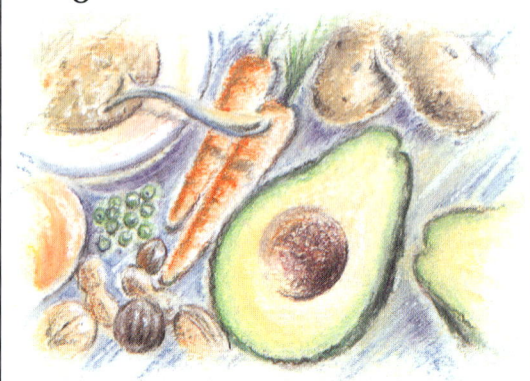

Nuts and seeds (proteins; polyunsaturated fats; magnesium; phosphorus; copper; potassium; selenium; zinc; B complex vitamins);
Wholegrains and cereals (proteins; carbohydrates; chromium; magnesium; manganese; phosphorus; potassium; selenium; B complex vitamins);
Potatoes and carrots (carbohydrates; vitamin A; folic acid; vitamin E);
Avocados (polyunsaturated fats; carbohydrates; vitamin A; folic acid; vitamin C; iron; magnesium; phosphorus; potassium);
Green vegetables – especially broccoli; beans and peas (carbohydrates; vitamin A; vitamin B6; folic acid; paba; vitamin C; vitamin E; calcium; iron);
Fruit – all varieties (carbohydrates; vitamin A; vitamin C);
Liver – preferably organic (protein; vitamin A; B vitamins; folic acid; vitamin D; vitamin E; copper; iron; phosphorus; potassium; zinc);
Fish, shellfish and seaweed (protein; vitamin A; B vitamins; vitamin D; calcium; copper; fluoride; iodine; iron; magnesium; phosphorus; selenium; sodium; sulphur; zinc).

Allergies and Food Intolerance

An allergy to a certain food can give many of the signs and symptoms of stress and it is widely believed that stress itself can result in an intolerance to a variety of foods. There are various signs that may suggest that you have a food allergy:

▪ history of allergies as a child – to milk or eggs, for example, (with age the body may adapt to a certain food, but under stress the allergy can recur);

▪ family history of allergies: hayfever, for example, or reactions to dust, cats or certain foods;

▪ rapid onset of symptoms after meals, with the symptoms fading slowly after a while;

▪ symptons disappear with anti-histamine preparations;

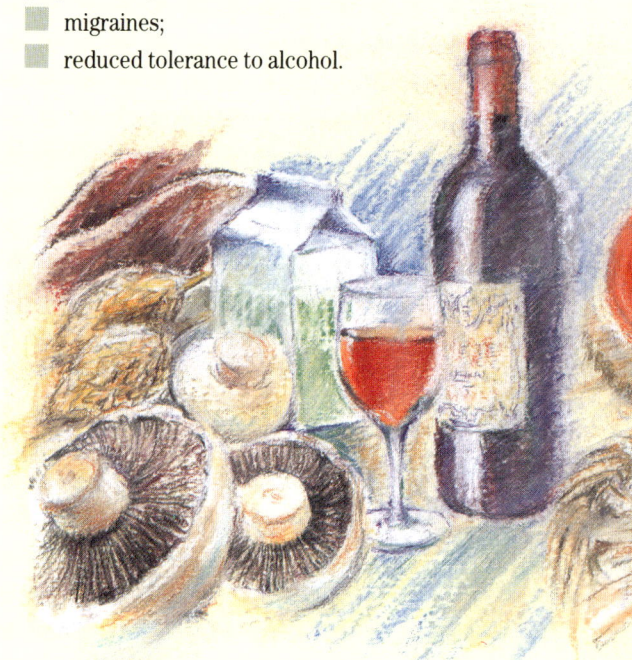

▪ migraines;

▪ reduced tolerance to alcohol.

You can be allergic to any food, but there are certain foods that seem to have a higher 'allergy factor' than others. These include:
wheat, rye, maize, milk, eggs, beef, fish and shell-fish, nuts, chocolate, sugar, coffee, tea, tomatoes, alcohol (especially red wines and port), yeast and all preservatives and colourings. It is also possible to be allergic to the mould that grows on many foods – common symptoms caused by this type of allergy include headaches and frequent colds. Mould can develop on any food, but is possible to cut the worst offenders out of your diet – these include cheese, beer, wine, and mushrooms. Be sure that nuts, whole grains, and oils are stored in airtight containers to keep them from going rancid.

While it is difficult to identify an allergy at home – it can be done with time and patience.

First, try to exclude all the foods that appear to cause reactions such as stomach ache, headaches, dizziness, fatigue or irritability soon after eating, for at least three weeks. Meanwhile, be careful to eat a balanced diet. If you feel better on this diet reintroduce the foods you have eliminated, one food at a time: if you are still allergic to the food you will notice the same symptoms as before – either within a few hours or within two to three days. For this reason, introduce new foods at about three-day intervals. If you suspect one food, stop eating it again for a while and retest later when you have worked through the other foods.

Some specialists recommend rotating foods, that is varying your intake on a daily basis so that, for example, you do not eat the same breakfast cereal every morning but rather every fourth morning, replacing cereals with fruit or protein breakfasts on the days in between.

It is sensible to attempt a non-allergic or elimination diet with the guidance of a qualified specialist. Ask your doctor to refer you to a reputable allergist or clinical ecologist.

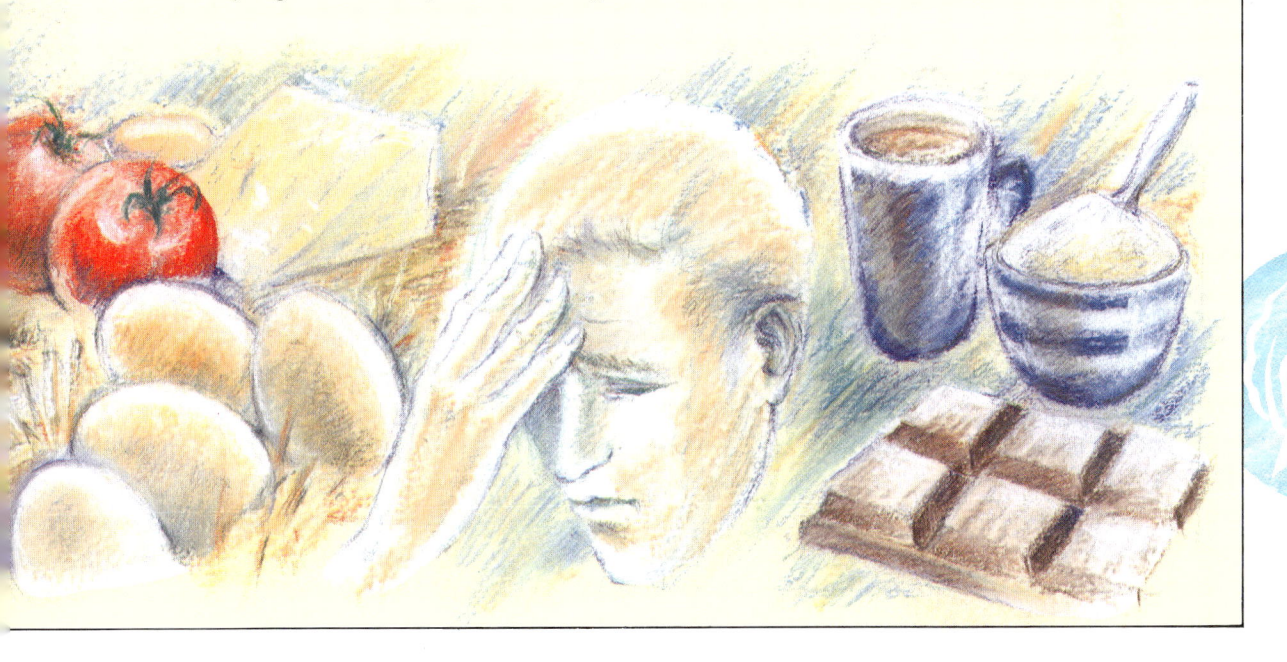

TECHNIQUES

NATUROPATHY

A system of care derived from the teachings of Hippocrates, the Greek physician and so-called founder of medicine, who believed that health depends on a balance between sleep, exercise and food. Naturopathy developed as an alternative form of medicine in the 19th century, when a number of people – not all of them doctors – began to advocate fresh air, pure water and plain food as a way of encouraging the body's own healing abilities. One of these was Harry Benjamin who laid down the fundamental principles of naturopathy in his 1936 work *Everybody's Guide to Nature Cure*; these still hold today.

The first emphasis of naturopathy is on the prevention of disease rather than its cure; naturopaths aim to assist the body's own power to maintain and restore health rather than treat a specific illness. All forms of disease, they believe, are the result of an accumulation in the body of toxins or waste products, this occurring 'through years of wrong habits of living'. According to the second principle of naturopathic healing, the body is always striving to maintain health, and symptoms of all acute diseases – from fever to typhoid – are the result of its attempts to throw off toxic waste materials that have accumulated to the point where they interfere with normal functioning. For example, one prime cause of a lack of balance in mind or body, of course, is stress.

Benjamin's third principle is that 'the body contains within itself the power to bring about a return to that condition of normal well-being known as health,

MEDICAL ALERT

Remember that naturopathy does not attempt to *cure* disease, and should not be used as a treatment for any serious medical problems. Its aim is to prevent disease, by maintaining the body's natural balances and reducing stress.
If you are taking any prescribed drugs, do not start a cleansing mono-diet or a juice-diet before consulting your doctor.

Method

You can put some of the basic naturopathic principles into practice by yourself – though it is probably better to visit an experienced naturopath if you can. Evaluate your own lifestyle: when and where do you feel stress, and why? Do you get adequate rest and recreation? Do you eat well and healthily, or do you rely on fast food?

1 Write down a realistic, ideal lifestyle – naturopaths are realists and realize that too drastic a change is impossible to maintain. Try to strike a balance between rest, fresh air, exercise and work, and combine this with good nutrition.

2 As a trial, to see how naturopathy might suit you, try a mono-diet or a semi-fast over a weekend, or at any time when you are not under pressure. Do not use either of these diets for any longer than two days.
■ Mono-Diet: eat only grapes, bananas or grapefruits for two days. Grapefruit is good for reducing high levels of cholesterol.
■ Juice Diet: drink as much vegetable and/or pure fruit juice as you wish. If you suffer from diarrhoea as a result, stop.
■ On either diet drink lots of pure water to flush out the toxins. Sometimes these diets can cause bad breath – this is a sign that toxins are leaving the body. Try to drink more water to help the process. Do not drink any alcohol, tea or coffee.

3 Having rested the body by the use of a cleansing diet, you can start to adjust your regime for the future:
■ Try to cut down on cigarettes, alcohol and caffeine products – if possible cut them out altogether.

provided the right methods are employed to enable it to do so'. Benjamin proposed five 'right methods' to enable the body to recover: fasting; scientific dieting; hydrotherapy; general body-building; hygienic measures; and psychotherapy. Naturopaths vary in their interpretation of these measures but all practitioners will take a very detailed case history of a patient, including a family history, notes on lifestyle, likes and dislikes, eating habits and stress-inducing factors, as well as detailed observations of the patient's physical appearance – general demeanour, posture, breathing, brightness of eyes, complexion and so on.

The naturopath may prescribe a course of treatment, but it is the patient's responsibility to follow this – no drugs are involved, though some practitioners use homoeopathic or herbal remedies to stimulate the body's own healing systems. Naturopaths believe that healing illness with orthodox medicine merely suppresses symptoms, so that they are bound to reappear when the body is under stress. Many treatments start with a fast or semi-fast; this gives the body a rest and enables it to flush out any toxins and restore homoeostasis – the self-regulating mechanism of the body's own immune system – as well as giving over-worked digestive systems a time to recover. Fasting has been observed by the British naturopath, Leon Chaitow, as the oldest therapeutic method known. Perhaps the most important naturopathic treatment, though, is a balanced, high-fibre, wholefood diet, without chemical additives or foods that might have been in contact with pesticides or other poisonous chemicals during its manufacture.

■ Eat only additive-free food and cut down on red meat and dairy products. Eat wholemeal bread – not merely 'brown' bread, since in many cases this is merely dyed; wheatgerm bread is not the same as wholemeal bread.

■ Do not eat last thing at night as this puts a strain on your digestive system and often leads to insomnia – food eaten last thing at night is not metabolized by the body in the same way as that eaten during the day, and more of it is turned into fat. The old adage that one should breakfast like a king, lunch like a prince and dine like a pauper is good dietary and health advice.

■ Set time aside for exercise – half an hour, three times a week either at home or, preferably, in fresh air. Walk to work or the shops, for example, rather than taking a car or bus. Take a walk at lunch time or go for a swim.

■ By eating well and taking regular exercise, the body becomes more relaxed and sleep becomes deeper. This lowers stress levels and helps general relaxation. Once the body is more relaxed the problems that are producing stress often fall into perspective and seem more easily resolved.

Diet-Related Problems

Insomnia Avoid caffeine-rich foods and drink, such as coffee, tea, dark chocolate and cola.
Headaches Certain foods can trigger a headache or migraine: chewing gum, ice cream, monosodium glutamate, yellow food colourings and yeast. Avoid them all, or test one at a time to see whether it affects you. Other foods and drinks can cause a migraine: beer, red wine, coffee, tea, beans, cheese, chocolate, cured food – hot dogs, smoked fish, bacon and pork, for example; yoghurt and yeast extract.
Colitis, or Irritable Bowel Syndrome Triggers can be milk, wheat, eggs, nuts, tomatoes, onions, potatoes and smoked or fried foods. Bran helps to prevent the problem.
Ulcers Aspirin, coffee, alcohol, salt, spices and smoking can all be triggers. Cook with olive oil or polyunsaturated vegetable oils instead of butter.

HERBALISM

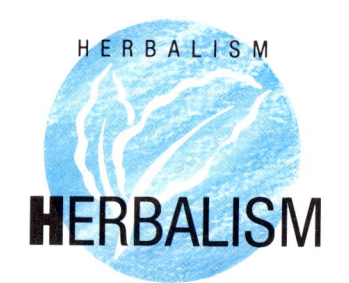

Records of using plants as medicines exist from as long ago as 3,000 BC, though advantage has probably been taken of the curative powers of plants for as long as humankind has existed. Before chemistry emerged as a science and synthetic drugs became available, the speciality we now call medical pharmacology was, for all practical purposes, herbalism.

The whole plant is used to prevent and cure disease. This is different from the technique of isolating plant-based drugs – the treatment of heart problems, for example, with digitalis, derived from the foxglove – since in such cases the active ingredient is extracted from the plant. Herbalists believe that this is a mistake, and that plants contain ingredients that both enhance the effect of the active ingredient and reduce any side-effects.

Herbalists take a holistic approach to medicine, treating the whole body, rather than specific symptoms of the disease. Like many other alternative therapists, they aim to stimulate the body's own defence systems and 'life-force' to combat disease. Of course, herbal treatments can have a profound effect on symptoms, but this is not the primary aim of therapists: the object is to restore and maintain the body's inherent and natural balance. As a result, herbalism is a very personalized therapy: each remedy has a different effect on each individual, both in terms of its potency and how it is ingested, whether by mouth, inhalation or rubbing into the skin. The efficacy of herbal remedies varies too, depending on where, when and how it was prepared.

Today, about 350,000 species of plants have been identified, but as yet the medicinal properties of only 10,000 or so are known. But as more and more people around the world come to rely on herbal remedies to cure disease, rather than use pharmaceutical drugs, and with the failure of modern medicine to 'cure' many chronic diseases as well as the horrific side-effects of some drugs, there has been a tremendous revival of interest in herbalism. The World Health Organisation is at present encouraging research into herbal remedies and their use in the Third World.

WATCHPOINT

If you wish to see a herbalist it is imperative that you go to a professionally registered practitioner, who will have received a rigorous training in plants and their uses and usually prepare their own remedies.

MEDICAL ALERT

Never exceed the suggested dose. Herbal remedies can have serious side-effects if taken incorrectly.

SELF-HELP

The aim of using herbal remedies for self-help purposes should be to use herbs which you personally find improve your general health. There are a number of possible remedies to suit any problem, and you will have to find out which is the most effective for you by trial and error. Many plant remedies are available over the counter in herbal shops, health food shops and in some chemists, but it is generally best to buy from the herbalist so that you may take advantage of his or her experience and seek advice on the most suitable herbs for your specific complaint. Always start with a single remedy, and seek advice as to how long to wait for improvement before trying another.

Remedies

Herbal remedies can be very effective in the treatment of symptoms of stress and in aiding relaxation. This list gives just a few of the many remedies available.

Camomile – diarrhoea; migraine; gastritis; colitis; over-indulgence in food or drink; insomnia; nightmares.
Valerian – insomnia; anxiety; tension.
Sage – insomnia; depression; increased perspiration; bad breath.
Garlic – high blood pressure; reduced resistance to infection.
Lemon Balm – anxiety; stress; palpitations.
Peppermint – indigestion; colic; anxiety.
Ginseng – stress; lack of energy; tiredness.
Rosemary – nervous tension; headaches.

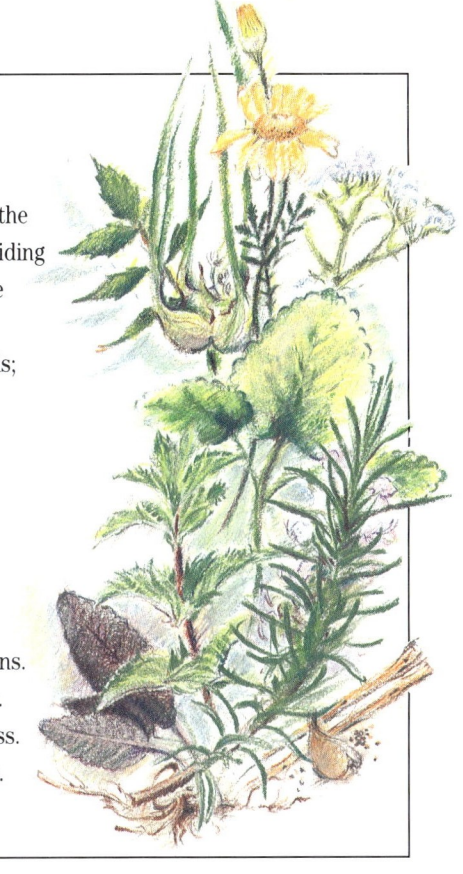

MEDICAL ALERT

Certain herbal preparations should never be taken during pregnancy, or if you have diabetes or a heart condition. Check with a herbalist if you have an existing medical condition, before using specific herbs. If you are taking any prescribed drug, it is essential that you check with your doctor before taking herbal remedies, since they can interact with drugs with possible harmful side-effects or reduce the drug's efficacy.

Method

There are as many ways to use herbs internally as there are externally.

1. If you have a digestive disturbance it is preferable to avoid taking by mouth and instead use herbs in the bath, as poultices or creams, or inhale the essential vapours of herbs put into boiling water.

2. Herbs can also be gargled, or massaged into the gums in a powdered form. Ask your herbalist how to prepare these external applications.

3. For taking herbs by mouth, prepare a herbal infusion by pouring a pint of boiling water over an ounce of dried herb or ground-up root (or 30 g in 0.5 l); leave to steep in a covered vessel for 5 to 15 minutes, and take by the cupful 1 to 3 times a day according to instructions.

4. You can also take herbs in syrup or tincture formulations, or in capsules available from the herbalist.

EVENING PRIMROSE OIL

A recent article in *World Medicine* asked what it is that schizophrenia, Parkinson's disease, eczema, alcoholism, obesity, rheumatoid arthritis, cardiovascular disease, breast disease, brittle nails, and premenstrual syndrome have in common? 'What links the maladies in this apparently random collection is that all respond to, or might in theory respond to, treatment with an oil extracted from the seeds of the evening primrose plant?' Although not entirely conclusive, the results of research on the above-mentioned disorders and with multiple sclerosis are promising.

TECHNIQUES

HOMOEOPATHY

Homoeopathy is a 200-year-old medical system you can use at home to treat a wide variety of acute health problems brought about by stress. The medicines or 'remedies' are natural substances, chosen from the animal, mineral and plant kingdom. The key to understanding homoeopathy is that no two people suffer from exactly the same problem. We each have our own highly individual ways of reacting to the stresses of life and of maintaining our inner harmony. Take as an example a simple headache. One person may find marked relief from taking warm drinks which would make another feel much worse; one may feel feverish and want fresh air while someone else might only wish to lie down. By taking a good look at your 'symptom picture', as explained in the following pages, you will be able to match up your 'guiding symptoms' with the best remedy for relieving them. The correct, individually suited homoeopathic medicine (see Selected Remedies) will stimulate your body's defenses rather than simply suppressing symptoms.

The originator of the technique was CFS Hahnemann, a physician, chemist and prolific scientific writer in the early 19th century. By his mid-thirties, Hahnemann had become so disillusioned by the appallingly brutal treatments that physicians inflicted on their patients that he resigned his job and devoted the rest of his life to trying to produce remedies that had no side-effects and were pain-free.

Hahnemann's first experiment was on himself; he had noticed that workers who harvested Peruvian bark (*cinchona*) often suffered from similar symptoms to people who had malaria. Putting this observation together with the fact that Peruvian bark was collected in order to produce quinine, with which malaria was treated, he formed a hypothesis that like might well cure like, and tested this by chewing *cinchona*. Within a few days, Hahnemann had all the symptoms of malaria; when he stopped taking *cinchona*, though, the symptoms disappeared.

Hahnemann's discovery that chewing less and less cinchona bark reversed the symptoms of malaria until he was restored to health led to a fundamental rule of treatment – The Law of Similars – which states that a remedy can cure a disease if it produces in a healthy person symptoms similar to the disease.

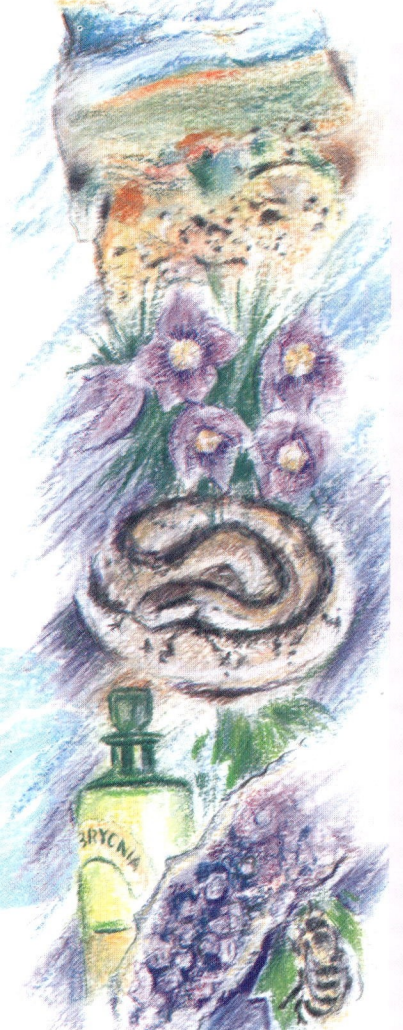

MEDICAL ALERT

Homoeopathic remedies should be used for self-help relief of short-term or acute symptoms only. If your symptoms persist or if your problem is chronic, such as a history of migraine headache, consult your medical doctor or a homoeopathic physician. Allergic reactions to homoeopathic remedies are uncommon, but consult your conventional medical doctor in the event of any major symptoms.
It is also a good idea to consult a homoeopathic practitioner who is familiar with the treatment.

QUICK ACTION

Specific remedies (when correctly chosen), can be relied upon to bring swift relief of certain acute symptoms: use arnica for shock, and first-aid emergencies; belladonna for a sudden bursting headache; chamomilla for great irritability and oversensitiveness; ignatia for anger and disappointment.

To avoid the unpleasant side-effect caused by triggering symptoms of the disease, he began to dilute the dosage considerably and not only found that the diluted remedy was just as good as the full-strength version, but often more effective. He called this process 'potentization'.

Hahnemann performed the dilution – and his methods are still used today – by mixing the ingredient with alcohol and water. The mixture was left to steep for at least a month, so that what he called the 'imprint' of the ingredient could be taken up by the liquid. It was then filtered several times and the end product – known as the 'mother tincture' – was then shaken vigorously, or 'successed', for several seconds to allow the 'imprint' of the original ingredient to be taken up by the whole contents. This process seemed to improve the potency of the remedy still further.

In further tests, Hahnemann gave various substances, some of them highly poisonous, such as snake venom, to volunteers – he called them 'provers' – so that he could match the signs and symptoms they produced to those of known diseases and test their efficacy as cures for those diseases. Soon, Hahnemann had a repertoire of nearly 100 remedies; by the end of the 19th century nearly 1,000 remedies were known; and today there are around 3,000 remedies.

Hahnemann came to believe that the correct remedy could only be found after a detailed history was taken of

Selected Remedies

Take your symptom picture as explained on p140, determine your key symptoms and match them up with the symptoms listed below to come up with the appropriate remedy. For example, if it is fear or panic that loom largest between you and relaxation, aconite would be the first remedy to try. If you feel fearful and have an upset stomach as well, you might choose *Arsenicum album*, since this addresses both symptoms equally.

Aconite – fear; panic; anxiety; shock; breathlessness; palpitations.
Aurum – depression.
Arnica – physical exhaustion; muscular aches and pains.
Arsenicum album – *exhaustion; restlessness; fear; upset stomach; nausea and diarrhoea.*
Belladonna – sudden fever and sweating; shaking; neuralgic pain that appears and disappears.
Byronia – irritability; headache; migraine.
Carbo Vegetabilis – hangover; indigestion; exhaustion.
Coffea – tension; restlessness; insomnia.
Gelsemium – nervousness; apprehension.
Nux vomica – irritability; impatience; quarrelsome tendencies; over-indulgence in food or drink; trifling ailments that assume too great an importance; emotional outbursts.
Pulsatilla – changeable emotions; tearfulness; shyness; public timidity and private aggression; menopause.
Silicea – anxiety with sweating and palpitations; lassitude.
Spigelia – timidity; sadness; palpitations; inability to concentrate.

both the problem presented and a patient's lifestyle, emotional state, personal preferences and family history. When knowledge of these factors was applied to the choice of a remedy, the patient's symptoms often worsened for a while – this showed that the correct remedy had been chosen – before the disease improved.

Homoeopathic hospitals soon began to open all over the world – in Britain, homoeopathy was given a boost when it was revealed that 84 per cent of the patients in the London Homoeopathic Hospital during the cholera epidemic of 1854 had survived, compared with 48 per cent in other hospitals.

Since then, Hahnemann's original methods have been refined and extended, in particular by Dr Constantine Hering and James Kent. The former formulated 'The Law of Cure', which states that a disease is cured from the inside out and downwards – from important internal organs to lesser organs and thus to the skin and from the centre of the body to the arms or legs. As a result, a successful treatment might increase the severity of symptoms for a short time, and as the body heals itself a disease might start to show itself on the patient's skin.

Kent further diluted Hahnemann's remedies and gave more emphasis to the characteristics of a patient: a tall, slim, fiery red-headed person, for example, would be given a different remedy from that chosen for a timid, plump, fair-haired person – even though their symptoms were the same.

Method

Many health food shops and chemists sell homoeopathic remedies and as these have no side-effects when taken in the correct doses, they are ideal self-help treatments. They should keep indefinitely, but must be stored away from camphor (contained in toothpaste) and substances that have a strong smell, such as coffee and volatile oils; sunlight can also harm them. Never move a homoeopathic remedy from one container to another, as this might destroy its potency.

Before Choosing A Remedy

Look at your overall 'symptom picture'.

1. Take note of any marked emotional states just prior to and during the illness.
2. Look at your physical symptoms; are you exhausted, feverish, aching, coughing?
3. Decide which symptoms are most serious or limiting to your optimal functioning.
4. Try to choose a remedy that stands out as a nearly perfect match.
5. For home prescribing use the lower potencies: 6x, 6c, 12x, 12c.
6. Do not touch the remedy (to avoid contamination) but pour into the bottle cap, then tip directly into the mouth and allow to dissolve under the tongue.
7. Avoid coffee, and products containing camphor, mint or menthol, during the treatment and for 48 hours afterwards; take remedies 20 minutes apart from food or drink.
8. If symptoms are intense you can repeat the dosage every ten to 15 minutes, if mild every one to four hours. Stop when better.
9. Should symptoms reappear after some improvement, repeat the dosage but for no more than two to three days. If the remedy does not work, reassess the key symptoms at this point and select another remedy.
10. Use one remedy at a time. Allow 24 hours for results before choosing another. Stop after you have tried two or three remedies without success.

Bach Flower Remedies

Devised in the 1920s by Dr Edward Bach, a pathologist and bacteriologist at University Hospital, London, this system of natural remedies uses wild flowers to heal the deep-seated negative emotional states that he believed were the cause of many diseases. Bach theorized that there are seven different emotional conditions: depression, despair, fear, uncertainty, indecision, over-concern for others and lack of interest in the present. These remedies were rarely used in the treatment of physical symptoms, unless Bach believed that they had, in fact, been caused by stress.

Bach began a search for flower remedies, believing that the dew collected from certain flowers could have remedial properties. Bach realized that it would be impractical to collect dew from flowers, so soaked them in pure spring water instead. He chose flower essences by holding his hand over a flowering plant: Bach would experience in himself the properties or 'aura' of the plant. In other words, if he was worried, holding his hand over flowers enabled him to find the one appropriate to that worry and its symptoms.

Bach further sub-divided each emotional state into different types, for each one of which there is a specific flower remedy, 38 in all. Mimulus, for example, can be used to treat a fear of known things; while aspen deals with a fear or apprehension of unknown origin. The remedies work in two ways: first, the specific remedy stimulates the body's own healing processes and encourages them to combat the negative state; second, it restores the body's equilibrium, so ridding it of the symptoms of stress or disease. Dr Bach was ridiculed by the medical profession during his lifetime, but today many medical practitioners find that his remedies can be as effective in the treatment of stress-related problems as pharmaceutical drugs; furthermore, they have no known side-effects or dangers. Dr Bach's intention was that people can bring about their own healing.

Method

A list of all Bach's remedies and the methods of treatment required can be found at most health shops. Generally, the remedies are bought in a concentrated form and are drunk after placing two drops in a glass of water or fruit juice; in an unconcentrated form, four drops can be placed on the tongue and swallowed.

Dr Bach produced one remedy called 'the Rescue Remedy', which he developed to reassure, comfort and calm – particularly in situations of unusual stress, such as a house move, a divorce, bereavement or redundancy. The rescue remedy is a mixture of five flowers and can be used in liquid or cream form.

QUICK ACTION

Take 4 to 8 drops of rescue remedy by mouth for a measure of immediate relief in cases of panic, sorrow, shock, terror, sudden bad news or accidents.

TECHNIQUES

COLOUR THERAPY

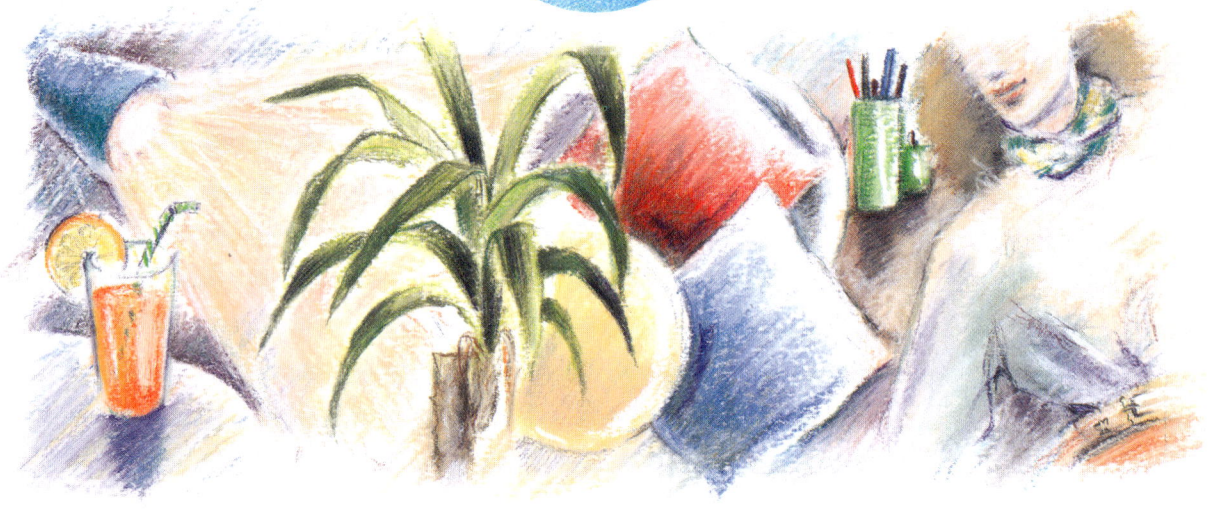

The importance of colour in healing was recognized by both the ancient Egyptians and classical Greeks – so much so that Egyptian temple complexes included a 'colour hall' where colour was used as a medical treatment. Colour therapy has always been one of the main weapons employed against disease by Ayurvedic Indian practitioners, too, the others being herbalism, naturopathy and meditation.

Although colour therapy is an ancient art, there was no real attempt to explain the scientific reasoning behind it until Dinshah P Ghadiali, a Hindu scientist, wrote a book called *The Spectro-Chrometry Encyclopaedia* in 1933. Ghadiali claimed that different colours vibrate at different rates, and that since each cell and organ of the body vibrates at its own rate in good health – the rate changing in ill-health – colour can 'reset', as it were, incorrect vibrations in the body.

At first sight, this concept may seem a little far-fetched. However, there is a considerable amount of circumstantial scientific evidence to support it. Light is a form of energy transmitted by the sun within a fixed span (or waveband) of frequencies, the whole range of frequencies being known as the electro-magnetic spectrum, that stretches from radio waves through X-rays to cosmic radiation. The span of frequencies over which light is transmitted can be subdivided into smaller frequency ranges, which represent individual colours (photographers refer to these frequencies as 'colour temperatures'); the effect can most easily be seen when light is passed through a prism, or in a rainbow – in both cases white light is divided into its components. At either side of the span of light frequencies on the electro-magnetic spectrum are two types of energy emission – 'invisible' light, one might say – that are used to heal, with great success, in conventional medicine: infra-red radiation, at the lower end of the span, and ultra-violet radiation, at the higher end. So it is likely that colour therapy can work – even if not necessarily for the reasons promoted by Ghadiali.

A number of experiments have been carried out to test the effects of colour on physical and mental well-being, and on concentration and performance. Research results from New England, in the United States, have shown that colour has an effect on blood pressure: after 30 minutes of exposure to blue light, blood pressure dropped; after the same time in red light, blood pressure rose. Many people could lower their blood pressure for a moment or two just by visualizing the colour blue.

Curiously, it does not seem necessary actually to see the colour, since blind people can achieve the same effect. Blind people, in particular, can often recognize colour by touch – the ability for eyeless sight being known as bio-introscopy. This is probably because an aura – an electro-magnetic field of colour vibrations, which blind people, in particular, can sense – surrounds all matter, animate and inanimate, as has been demonstrated by means of a technique called Kirlian photography. The aura surrounding the human body contains two bands: an inner band that outlines the body, and an outer, less distinct band that fades outwards. This aura can change from day to day, and even from minute to minute, depending on physical and mental health. Colour therapists believe that where there is any disharmony in the body, and especially stress, the colour in the inner band becomes discoloured and breaks up.

By examining a patient's aura in a Kirlian photograph, a colour therapist makes a diagnosis. The treatment then prescribed relies on a concept borrowed from Eastern medicine: that of *chakras*. In the West it is more or less common ground that there are three states, or components, of existence, these being the physical, the intellectual and the emotional. Eastern medicine, though, holds that there are seven states – the *chakras* – and that these have entry points to the body in the spine and head.

The *chakras* respond to vibrations from outside the body (including those of different colours) and pass them on to the different areas of the body through a network of links between them. Each *chakra* absorbs a different one of the seven colours that comprise the rainbow; the colour, and the *chakra* to which it is applied, depending on the nature of the patient's problem.

This is very much the technical side of colour therapy, whose use is complex and depends on considerable training in the techniques. It is possible, though, to use some of the principles of colour therapy to relieve stress and aid relaxation; in fact, it is fascinating to see how many of the healing tenets of colour have become lodged in our daily lives, our perceptions and even our language. Just think of a peach-coloured room with a crackling fire of red and orange: it appears welcoming and relaxing; a room without any sunlight, though, decorated in sombre greys and blues feels cold and remote. We even ascribe different emotions to different colours: we say that someone is 'in the pink', for example, 'green with jealousy', 'red with rage' and so on. Everyone has a favourite colour, too: studies have shown that blue is by far the most popular, with red second; yellow seems to be the least popular colour of all.

Method
At home

1. Use tinted light bulbs with warm-coloured shades in your living-room and bedroom.

2. When redecorating, think of using earth colours – peaches, pinks, greens and warm blues.

3. Never decorate a sunless room in a dark or cold colour – to do so will make the walls crowd in and produce a feeling of claustrophobia. If you do use such colours, compensate by filling the room with warm light.

4. Replace strip-lighting at home with softer lighting.

5. Use plants and flowers to add colour and life to a drab room.

6. Add food colouring to your bathwater – green and blue to relax, or orange and red to stimulate.

7. Use vivid coloured cushions to brighten a dull room.

8. Try to make sure that at least one room in your house has a decor that is relaxing and soothing – make use of this space when you feel depressed, or when trying out the various therapies in this book.

On the move

1. Go for a walk in the country or a park – this is especially useful when you're feeling low. Look at the sky, enjoy the differing sensations of sunshine or wind on your face; notice the various shades of colour and light all around you and try to let them soak into you.

2. When setting off on a long car journey, try to plan your route so that you travel at least part of the way on minor or scenic roads, taking in attractive towns and beauty spots. Take notice of the subtle differences in colours and hue as you pass.

3. Plan your route to work so that you walk for at least part of the way – through a park, along a river bank or through gardens. Look for window boxes full of flowers, the first blossoms of spring or the russet and orange hues of autumn.

At the office

1. If your office is lit by strip-lighting, ask whether it can be changed: the light is produced in flashes so close together that they seem continuous; nevertheless, they do produce tension on a sub-conscious level. If it is not possible to change strip-lighting, try to position yourself so that the light does not glare straight down at you – the glare from bright lights, especially when reflected on white desks, causes the pupils of the eyes to constrict, which often results in a headache. Try placing a tinted light bulb in a desk lamp to reduce the glare from a white desk. On the other hand, a dim room

---

Colours and their Associations

All the following colours can be used in different shades: pastels are good for relaxation; darker colours have a more subduing effect; and the clearer, vivid colours have more clarifying qualities.

Red Stimulating, aggressive, strengthens will-power and stimulates vitality. Helpful in lethargy and depression, but use with caution, since this colour can be very powerful; always follow with exposure to blue to create harmony.

Orange Warm, suggests a sense of well-being and restores vitality. Used to treat negative feelings, insecurity, inertia, lassitude, odd aches and pains and muscular cramps.

Yellow Powerful and mentally stimulating. Helpful for depression, skin problems and mental lethargy.

Green Gives a sense of proportion and balance, restoring the body's natural harmony. Use to treat tension (especially headaches), stress, moodiness and over-emotional behaviour.

Blue Calming, relaxing and cleansing; symbolizes love and truth. Helpful in encouraging relaxation, especially when feeling irritable, jumpy or aggressive.

Indigo Cool and clarifying, restores a balance between the individual and the outside world. Used to treat obsessions and emotional instability.

Violet Harmonizes the body, mind and spirit. As ultra-violet, this colour is used in conventional Western medicine to treat skin conditions and to restore the body's natural balance of salts. Use at home to treat insomnia, over-sensitivity and tension.

Blue–Green These shades are particularly useful to promote relaxation and the release of tensions.

Pink Traditionally, the colour of love. Use it to create a feeling of warmth coupled with energy.

Peach/Apricot Warm and relaxing; ideal when you feel physically exhausted.

makes the pupils more enlarged, which can result in a feeling of fatigue. Make sure you have plenty of warm, bright light to work by.

2 Make sure that the accessories on your desk are in your favourite colours.

3 If you can, choose different posters and pictures to decorate your working area; choose vivid colours for those times when you feel depressed, and restful and soothing shades when you feel tense and irritable.

What you should wear

1 Choose your clothes according to their colour, to enhance or change your mood.

2 Either throw out drab, washed-out clothes or dye them another colour.

3 Liven up clothes with a colourful scarf, a tie, a belt or jewellery.

4 The next time you buy a coat, try to choose a colour that will cheer you up on a dull, grey day in the winter.

5 Experiment with different colours. Withdrawn, shy people often wear greys and browns: add a striking and contrasting scarf or shirt.

Irritable, noisy people tend to reds, black and oranges: contrast with turquoises, blues and greens.

Cold, over-controlled people generally wear blues, greys and blacks: warm your outlook with pinks, peaches and apricot.

Use colour creatively

1 Eat and drink foods and liquids of the colours you wish to emphasize: if you wish to become more outgoing, for example, try eating oranges and parsnips and drinking orange or carrot juice. Some therapists claim that a piece of coloured cellophane placed over a glass of water that is left in the sun for a few hours will imprint the water with that colour's energy properties – the concept is similar to that of homoeopathy and Bach Flower Remedies.

2 Swathe your body in an appropriate colour by fitting a coloured light bulb to a lamp; if you wish, ask at your health food shop for a special colour therapist's lamp. This comes with a variety of coloured lenses and filters.

3 Practise visualizing the colour that you need to change or enhance your mood. Most people find this difficult at first, but succeed with practice.

4 Try what is called 'colour breathing': either bathe yourself and the room in the colour of your choice, or visualize the colour, then relax and breathe deeply, holding your breath for a few seconds while you concentrate on the colour filling your body. Breathe out and repeat three or four times, then relax. Repeat this exercise three times or so a week.

Chakras

Each *chakra* responds to a rainbow colour, which can be used for healing at that point.

The Root (Etheric) Centre is at the base of the spine. Use red.
The Sacral (Emotional) Centre is at the small of the back, slightly to the left. Use orange.
The Solar (Lower Intellectual) Centre is at the mid-back, opposite the solar plexus. Use yellow.
The Heart (High Mental) Centre is between the shoulder blades opposite the heart. Use green.
The Throat (Spiritual) Centre is at the base of the skull. Use blue.
The Brow (Intuitional) Centre is at the centre of the brow. Use indigo.
The Crown (Absolute) Centre is on the dome of the head. Use violet.

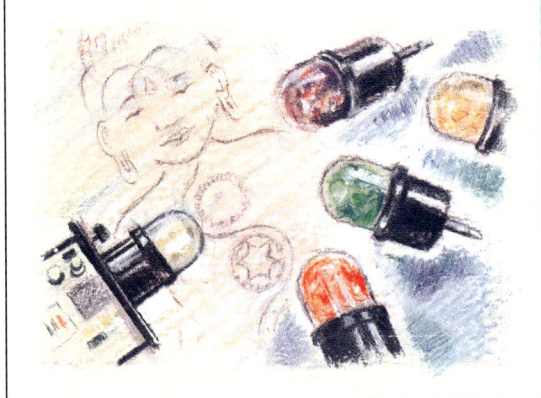

TECHNIQUES

CRYSTAL AND GEM THERAPY

Crystal and gem therapy is closely aligned with colour therapy and has a similar history to it. Gems and crystals have been treasured since the start of civilization, both for their beauty and colour and their inherent qualities and forces. Crystals, in particular, have been revered for centuries – both native Americans and Tibetans carried pouches containing crystals next to their skin.

Crystals are claimed to work in the same way as colours, by transmitting their energies to those who wear them in the form of vibrations. The healing forces of gems and crystals can be judged by their colour, and as for colour therapy, work on the *chakras*.

Method

Gem therapists say that one should not choose a stone or crystal, but let it choose you. When you come across a gem or crystal that has the power to help you, you will, somehow, know it. Gems need not be expensive, but plastic costume jewellery will not do. Look at various different stones, feel them, and choose the colour of stone that helps stress conditions best and aids relaxation following the same principles as those in colour therapy.

When you have found a colour and type of stone that feels right for you, try to buy more than one example. It may be worthwhile to buy gems in each of the seven colours, so that you can use different stones to help with different problems. Crystals are especially important for relaxation and are traditionally used during meditation, especially when placed over the sixth *chakra* between the brows (often referred to as the 'third eye').

Bear in mind that the blues, indigos, violets and greens are the most relaxing colours, while reds, corals, oranges and yellows tend to be stimulating and energizing.

Before you start any gem or crystal therapy, though, you must clean the stone in order to remove any impurities, since these can reduce effectiveness – wash it under running water for a few hours, or, preferably, leave it beneath a quartz crystal. Wait for a day before starting therapy. Gem and crystal therapy is a very personal technique, and what follows are merely guidelines. See which method works for you.

1 Hold the gem in the palm of your hand while relaxing (*see* Basic Relaxation Technique) and try to empty your mind of all thoughts. Visualize the vibrations of the stone entering your hand and moving around the body.

2 Place the appropriate stone on the relevant *chakra* for about 30 minutes – this may be a point on the spine or a spot on the front of the body, for example a green stone on the breast bone slightly to the left.

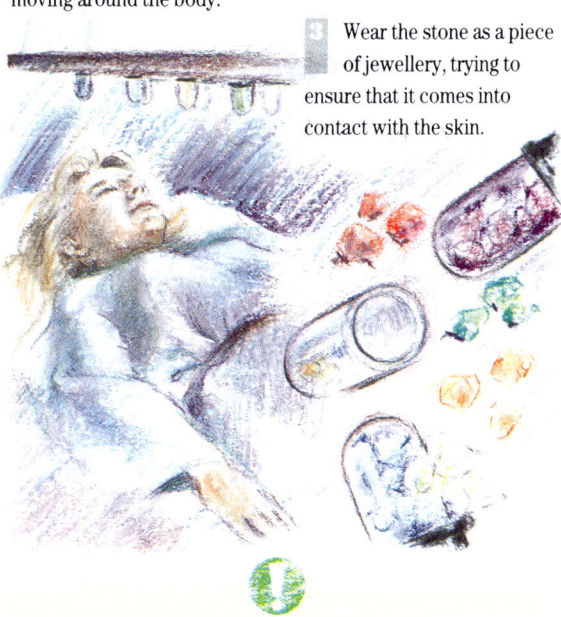

3 Wear the stone as a piece of jewellery, trying to ensure that it comes into contact with the skin.

WATCHPOINT

Look after the gems and clean them frequently. Leave them out in the sun when you can, so that they can renew their energies.

DANCE THERAPY AND EURHYTHMY

Ever since the dawn of civilization, dancing has been used to stimulate and relax, as a form of communication and of self-expression. Primitive people also used dance forms to unite their people and to achieve trance-like states for healing purposes. In medieval times dance was formalized into set routines that denied free expression, and this remained the fashion until the American dancer, Isadora Duncan, revolutionized the art in the early years of the 20th century, and greatly influenced the development of ballet and modern expressive dance. She both entranced and scandalized Europe with her 'free', bare-footed dancing, based on classical Greek forms, wearing a modified, diaphanous tunic and numerous scarves.

Another development in dance as therapy came in the 1920s from Rudolf Steiner, the father of a self-healing philosophy called 'anthroposophical medicine'. He created a dance movement that was linked to the sounds of speech, called eurhythmy, as part of his treatment for stress-related diseases and as an aid to relaxation. Later, medical practitioners realized the potential of dance therapy for unlocking repressed anger and emotion in the treatment of the mentally and emotionally disturbed, and today many mental hospitals employ full-time dance therapists.

Dancing is a highly personal activity that releases both physical and mental stress. There are no hard and fast rules about what to do, since what works for one person may not be right for another; but, in all cases, it can teach us a fuller awareness of ourselves. Dancing can release pent-up emotion, too, as well as tension and self-consciousness. Unfortunately, it is all too often only the young who dance without inhibition – adults tend to be over self-conscious about their abilities and primarily concerned with the image they are creating. In fact, nearly everyone can benefit from dance therapy – old and young, fat or thin, fit or unfit. Dancing has an extraordinary 'feedback' effect on the whole body, increasing sensation, stimulating the body's own pain-relieving hormones – the endorphins – and unlocking hidden tensions in the mind and body. The end result is a feeling of well-being and relaxation.

Method

1. Start by dancing on your own at home to any type of music that you like. Make sure you will not be disturbed – unplug the phone, lock the door and draw the curtains. Do not try to reproduce any formalized dance movement, but just allow your body to move naturally and easily in whatever way comes to you. Dance slowly to start with, in order to warm up your muscles, then follow the music and your feelings. Intersperse slow, flowing movements with bursts of physical activity.

2. Move as much of your body as you can, without straining – remember it's important that you enjoy what you're doing.

3. Try to dance for 15 minutes each day.

4. As you become less self-conscious, join a dance class or club; try dancing with a partner – but always remember you are primarily dancing for yourself, not to impress others.

5. Dance with your children – especially pre-school age children.

6. If you come home from work exhausted and depressed, play some lively music and dance around the house – this is much more effective than slumping in front of the television.

7. Buy a personal stereo so that you can dance anywhere and at any time – even a few minutes is beneficial.

8. Hire a dance video and dance along with the film and the music.

TECHNIQUES

MUSIC THERAPY

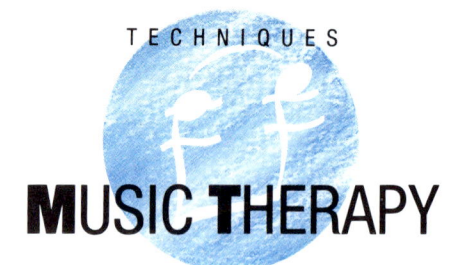

The healing powers of music have been recognized for centuries, and there are numerous stories about how they were once used. The belief was – and still is (*see* Sound Therapy) – that the cells of the body can vibrate at various rates, and that the symptoms of disease are the result of a variation in the rate of vibration that puts the affected organ or system out of harmony with the rest of the body.

Healers, it was believed, could somehow 'feel' the vibrations of a patient's cells, and by playing the appropriate note on an instrument could re-educate the cells, setting up vibrations at the correct rate, so curing the disease. Pythagoras, the classical Greek mathematician, it is said, played music of variable rhythms and melodic intervals in order to heal; Aristotle, the philosopher, used the flute to arouse strong emotions in the repressed; and it was common practice in ancient Greek society to play zither music to those affected by stomach problems.

But the use of music as a therapy is not just an ancient art. Hindu Indians have always used music to heal, by inducing relaxation and deepening meditation, while both Zen Buddhists in Japan and American Indians still employ atonal chanting to deepen trances. The keening or wailing of women at funerals is a traditional way of releasing emotion and stress, and national anthems and tribal songs still unify people by evoking a common response.

In Western society, though, it is only in this century that the healing power of music has been relearnt. Psychiatrists have found that soothing music helps in serious mental disorders; psychologists have discovered that music helps their patients to relax and release pent-up emotions; obstetricians have worked out that pulsating sounds in premature baby units increase an infant's chance of survival. There has been an overall increase in the use of music to heal, relax and promote well-being.

One problem with music therapy, however, is that though music can cross all barriers of class and race, its appreciation is still a matter of personal taste and tradition. Some research supports the theory that individual responses to rhythm and music are biologically determined by the external sounds heard within the womb, and by the sound of the maternal heartbeat and breathing.

Nevertheless, music is a powerful aid to self-expression and socialization. It can evoke different moods and feelings, increase vitality or induce

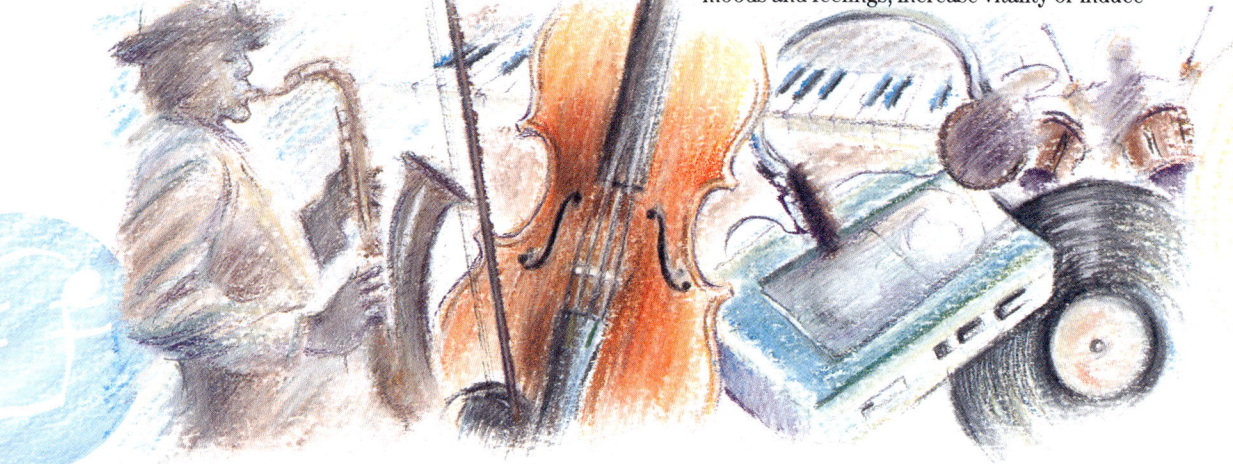

MUSIC

relaxation; it can also develop self-confidence and improve concentration. Composers of music hear tunes in their imaginations and transmit these images to listeners through the music, thereby suggesting to them colour, emotion and image. The listeners react to this information and feel sad or happy, revitalized, tense or relaxed according to the musical score.

Music affects both the right and left hemispheres of the brain. Vocals are assimilated in the left hemisphere and instrumental music in the right hemisphere. The right hemisphere controls emotion and the creative side of the mind, so to stimulate – as for depression – or to relax – as in stress – it is essential that one listens to the appropriate music. Research has shown, for example, that what is technically described as the 'anapestic stopped beat' often used in rock music can induce stress, while the more flowing rhythms of jazz and blues music can halt the downward spiral of many mental conditions, such as depression. Classical music, on the other hand, evokes different responses, according to the composer and the individual work, and how completely the emotions of the listener become involved.

Toning

There is tremendous interest in this technique. Toning involves singing at a very basic level: in fact, using sounds, such as grunts, sighs, 'ohs' and 'ahs' to rid yourself of inhibitions. You can visit a toning therapist, who will show you how to sing in this way, and sing along with you.

The theory behind toning is that people are inhibited from shouting and singing as we grow up, unless we do so as a release of aggression, and that this enforced silence prevents us from releasing our pent-up emotions and results in stress. By relearning the ability to shout, sing, hum and so on we can release these tensions before they become a problem. Singing can also act on the brain's pain-killing hormones, the endorphins, and so relieve pain. Try at home on your own: yell, keen (a screeching yell similar to that produced by an owl), grunt, hum and sing.

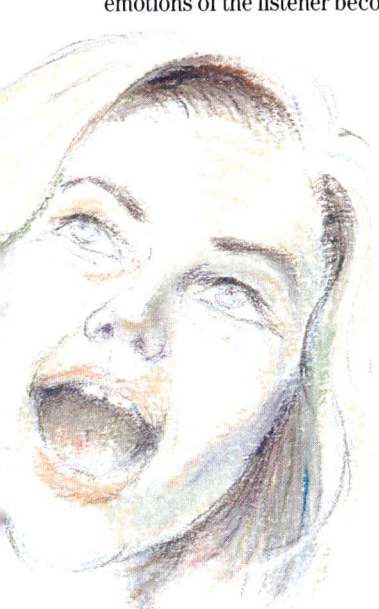

Method

1 Experiment in finding music that helps *you* to relax – whether a violin concerto, jazz, New-Age music, a ballad or the blues – and select music that revitalizes and makes you feel optimistic. Listen to your favourite pieces on a personal stereo with headphones – in the street, at the end of the day or at any time you feel in the need of relaxation or a pick-me-up.

2 Remember that your voice is a musical instrument, too; everyone can sing if they can speak. It does not matter if you are off-key or miss notes, because singing is a wonderful way of discharging feelings or giving yourself an uplift. Sing in the bath, in your car, around the house or on a walk. Keep a notebook in which you can write down the words to your favourite tunes, and sing along with the vocalist; try singing to your children if they are tired, tetchy or argumentative.

3 Take up a musical instrument – the piano and the guitar are reputed to be the most relaxing ones, but any instrument will do. Drums can be used to produce rhythm and to beat along in time to your favourite songs, and they help dispel aggression; or fill up milk bottles and beat out a tune on them with the spoons. Music can be produced from almost anything, so experiment.

TECHNIQUES

ART THERAPY

The use of art – drawing, painting, sculpture – as a means of self-expression and as a way of releasing hidden feelings and emotions is well-known. Unfortunately many people never attempt to draw or paint when they are grown up, believing that the ability to draw is an inborn talent, and that if they do not have the gift it would be frustrating and stressful to try to draw.

Yet, as children, most of us draw instinctively and naturally from a very young age, anywhere and on anything. When in a temper or frustrated, the furious squiggles, slashing shapes and thrown paint illustrate inherent ability in children to let go of their tension. In a calm, happy mood children tend to concentrate on pictures that depict their world, with smiling faces, animals and suns. As they grow, they start to portray what they feel through their images. Around the age of 10, children tend to grow out of the stage of intuitive composition and begin to strive for realism – sometimes losing the freedom of expression in their early pictures; many people never recapture this innate creativity. As a result, the grown-up child may well have lost an important outlet for pent-up emotions and subconscious feelings while stress levels increase. Like music, art can be used to express the emotional, imaginative, free and unconscious side of our personality, by utilizing form and colour to depict a positive atmosphere and feelings.

Art therapy is widely used in hospitals and schools, especially for the treatment of emotional problems and mental disturbance. Anyone can join an art course, or even a specialist art therapy course, as an ideal self-help treatment, for stress and relaxation. The equipment is cheap and easily available, can be carried around in a handbag or a briefcase and you can devote as much or as little time to the therapy as you wish. It does not matter if you cannot produce anything remotely like a work of art – the important thing is to express yourself in some way.

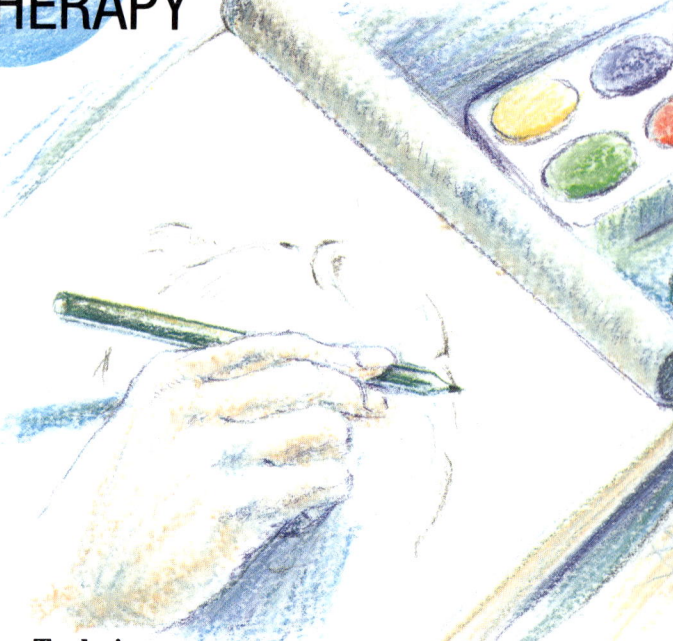

Techniques

To use art as a relaxation therapy, you need to be able to switch off the critical and objective side of your brain and allow the visual and subjective side to take control. Doing this, and allowing yourself to draw as freely and easily as you did as a young child, may take some practice. Try one of the other relaxation techniques first, such as meditation, to help get yourself in the right frame of mind. Art teachers do use one or two special techniques as follows, to help make the switch.

1 Place a well-known object – a portrait, for example, a telephone or a coffee pot – upside-down on a table in front of you. Upside-down is important, since this makes it more difficult for the objective side of your brain to label and recognize the object, so that you are more likely to draw what you see, rather than what you think you should be seeing. Use pencil on a large sheet of paper, and draw exactly what you see – don't use a rubber, or make any corrections. Draw as slowly as you can, losing consciousness of time, and concentrate solely on drawing what is in front of you: the shape and the texture. Don't worry if the

ART

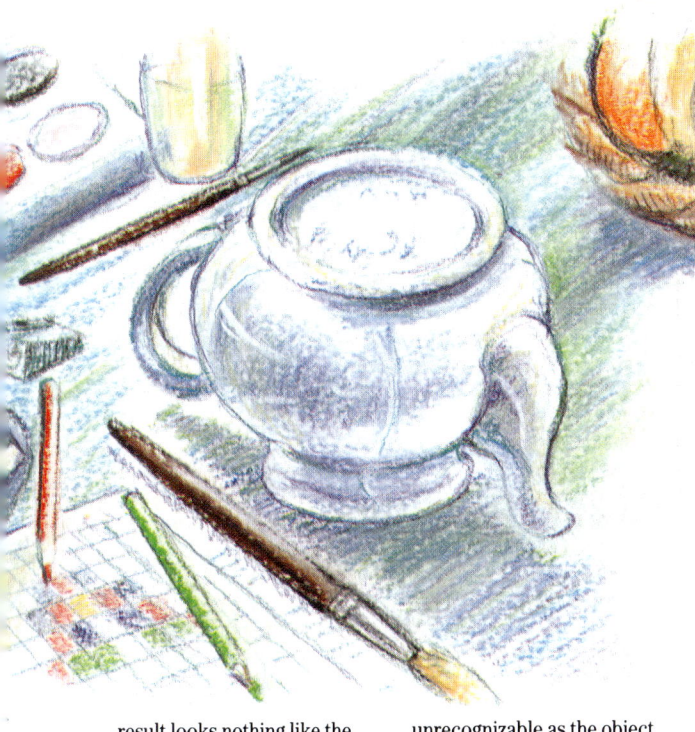

result looks nothing like the object – try not to examine the drawing too closely, but concentrate instead on the object itself.

2 Choose something fairly detailed and complicated to draw – a shoe, perhaps, or a bowl of fruit – and place it slightly away from you. Look at the object, rather than your drawing, all the while trying to visualize your hand as it draws what you can see. Visualize the lines on the paper as if they were an extension of the images that are travelling from the object to your brain. Again, be as slow as possible. Don't look at the object as a whole, but examine it bit by bit, taking in every curve, line, contour and edge. It may well be nearly unrecognizable as the object when you have finished, but resist the urge to change it or alter it in anyway. Repeat the exercise with other objects.

3 Conjure up a picture in your head before you put anything on paper. Fill in all the details in your mind. Is the weather hot or cold? Are there any people or animals in the scene? Are they happy or sad? Do not force the image – just let it come to you. Do not put something in because you think it would make a more pleasing composition. Then draw or paint the image that you hold in your mind, without changing it in any way. As you paint, focus on the picture in your head, not on what you are painting.

Method

Painting what you see is not the only way of using art in a therapeutic way.

1 Your signature is a form of art, and one that can say a lot about you. Look at your own signature – is it free and flowing or small and tight, legible or a squiggle? What does it tell you about yourself, and what does it tell other people about you? Try to sign your name in a number of different styles, as when you are relaxed, happy, angry, anxious and stressed. Look at the differences. If your signature is habitually 'tight' or 'hard', practise signing your name in a relaxed, flowing way. Every time you sign your name relax your hands beforehand; then let the signature flow from your pen. With practice you can change an 'uptight' signature into one that reflects a relaxed personality.

2 Keep a pencil and some paper always at hand. If someone upsets you, draw them – quickly and roughly, as a basic cartoon. Just a few lines will do. Then tear the drawing into small pieces and throw it away; you will feel the stress that the incident has caused you disappear with the pieces of paper.

3 Take a piece of graph paper and colour in the squares with crayons or felt-tip pens. Create a pattern, like a mosaic. Blank your mind out to anything else, and concentrate on the colours you are using and pattern you are forming.

4 Paint or draw if you feel tense at home. Set aside 30 minutes when you can be sure there will no distractions or interruptions. Draw or paint whatever you feel like – even if the result is not a picture but just random swirls of colour and shapes. Do not rush, or try to depict anything artistically; just let the picture form itself without any conscious thought. When using art therapy for relaxation, you are not trying to produce a work of art – though who knows? You may well find a hidden talent and real artistic merit.

TECHNIQUES

Pattern and Pyramid Therapy

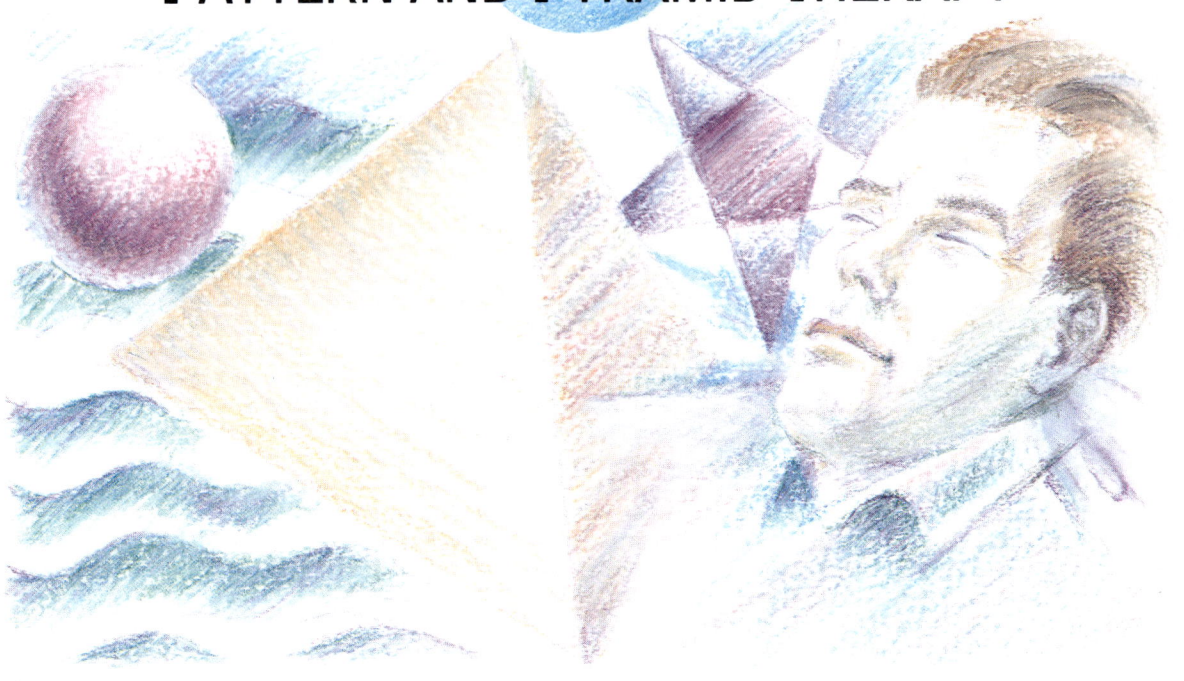

Pattern or pyramid therapy relies on the idea that shape can have an effect on a person's emotional and physical state. The ancient Babylonians and Egyptians certainly believed this to be true: they frequently used shape for healing purposes, and, of course, the Egyptains built the pyramids.

Today about 30 pyramids are still standing in Egypt – about a third of the number built originally. The Great Pyramid at Giza, the largest building ever constructed and equivalent in mass to about 30 of New York's Empire State Building, was completed in the Fourth Dynasty, between 2680 and 2565 BC, at the direction of Cheops (called Khufu by the Egyptians). This extraordinary construction is 146 m high (160 yd) and 230 m (251 yd) across. But it is not only the Great Pyramid's size that is remarkable, but its positioning and proportions: it is aligned exactly on true magnetic north, and stands precisely at the centre of the earth's land mass. As far as the proportions are concerned, the circumference of its base is the same as the circumference of a circle, whose radius is the height of the pyramid: such trigonometric exactitude could scarcely have occurred by chance.

It seems that the ancient Egyptians devised a shape and a set of proportions that have remarkable powers – so much so that all pyramids produced today for healing purpose are based on the Great Pyramid. Some researchers have shown that this shape has the ability to concentrate the earth's electromagnetic waves, and other types of energy that we do not fully understand. For example, Antoine Bovis, a French researcher, built a pyramid in the 1930s and found that the bodies of small animals, as well as fruit and vegetables became mummified when left in his pyramid.

At the time, Bovis's claims were ridiculed, but since then his experimental results have been replicated, and even stranger phenomena have been claimed. Among these have been the ability of pyramids to affect mood and emotions; to make plants inside them grow faster; to delay the process by which milk, for example, turns sour and a razor blade becomes blunt. It has been shown that a pyramid can increase the strength of the 'alpha' waves of the brain, which can help to increase concentration, diminish anxiety and hyperactivity, thus producing a feeling of relaxation and calm. Some people make extravagant claims for pyramids, saying that they can prolong youth and cure disease. Such claims have not been proven, and seem very unlikely.

The properties of pyramids have, then, to a certain extent been observed. But other shapes, and patterns, too, can have their effects on people, as builders and architects have long been aware: great buildings, for example cathedrals and mosques, all have their own atmosphere of harmony and tranquillity, and can impart this to the visitor. In fact, the basic principle that is used to create this harmony and symmetry was laid down by the Greek geometrician, Euclid, as long ago as 300 BC. He first described the set of proportions based on the Golden Ratio of height to width of 1:1.618033989. When this ratio is applied to a rectangle – the Golden Section – the resulting shape can be sub-divided into a square and another rectangle; this second rectangle has the same properties as the first one. The Golden Ratio and Golden Section have been used throughout the history of architecture, and have become so synonymous with the concept of civilization that their proportions have been inscribed on tablets carried by American space probes, as a means of communicating with other life forms in the solar system.

Yet it is not only the shape of buildings that affects our moods. Everyday objects can also have influence over our feelings, as manufacturers are only too aware. Much research is carried out to ensure that products are attractively shaped and carry patterns that help them sell: one recent study comparing the popularity of nine different shapes showed that a pentagram was by far the most popular, followed by a sphere and a wavy line; a straight line came last.

Amongst others, alternative therapists believe that surrounding oneself with shapes and patterns that are harmonious and, as with pyramids, that have their own particular power, helps to create the correct ambiance for good health – and, therefore for relaxation and the reduction of stress.

Method

1. See if it would be worthwhile, or possible, to move your work station to a better position – avoid sitting with your back to a sharp angle or a dark corner; this can often be strangely unsettling and make it difficult to relax. The Chinese, who place a lot of importance on shape, sometimes place a statue of a lion on their desks to ward off evil spirits – or a frog if the evil spirit is weak.

2. Check the arrangement of the furniture in your living-room and bedroom. Does it have a sense of proportion in its position in the room and its shape, or does it appear to be placed at random? See if you can give the room a more harmonious pattern by rearranging the furniture and the ornaments.

3. Avoid jagged shapes and hard lines, both in the patterns you wear and the decorations and furnishings of your home.

4. Visit a famous building that has stood the test of time, and try to sense the harmony of its external and internal proportions, and its sense of rightness, both in itself and in its relationship to the environment.

5. Consider buying a pyramid – ask at your local health food shop. Some people sleep beneath pyramid shapes; others relax quietly at home while contemplating a pyramid.

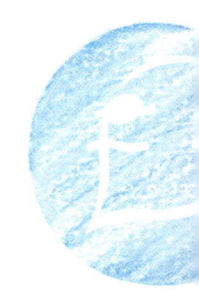

BIBLIOGRAPHY

Breaking the Stress Habit, Andrew G Goliszek, Carolina Press 1987

Coping with Stress: A Woman's Guide, Dr Georgia Witkin-Lanoil, Sheldon Press 1984

Coping with Stress, Donald Meichenbaum, Century Publishing 1983

Managing Stress: The practical guide to using stress positively, Ursula Markham, Element Books Limited 1989

Overcoming Stress, Dr Vernon Coleman, Sheldon Press 1988

The Relaxation Response, H Benson, Fontana 1977

The Serenity Principle: Finding Inner Peace in Recovery, Joseph V Bailey, Harper & Row Publishers 1990

Stress and Relaxation, Leslie Kenton, Portland House/Windward 1986

Stress Management, E Charlsworth, Corgi 1989

Stress without Distress, Hans Selye, Corgi Book 1975

Stresswise: a practical guide for dealing with stress, Dr Terry Looker & Dr Olga Gregson, Hodder & Stoughton 1989

Total Relaxation in Five Steps: The Alpha Plan, Louis Proto, Penguin Books 1989

Headaches: The Drugless Way to Lasting Relief!, Harry C Ehrmantraut, PhD, Celestial Arts 1987

No More Headaches, Lilian Rowen, Sheldon Press 1982

Chinese Massage Therapy: A handbook of therapeutic massage, Routledge & Kegan Paul Ltd 1983

The Complete Book of Massage, Clare Maxwell-Hudson, Dorling Kindersley 1988

Therapeutic Touch: A Practical Guide, Janet Macrae, Arkana 1987

Practical Aromatherapy: How to Use Essential Oils to Restore Vitality, Shirley Price, Thorsons 1987

Acupressure for Women, Cathryn Bauer, The Crossing Press 1987

Acupressure Techniques: a self-help guide, Dr Julian Kenyon, Thorsons 1987

How to Heal Yourself using Foot Acupressure, Michael Blate, Routledge and Kegan Paul 1983

How to Heal Yourself using Hand Acupressure, Michael Blate, Routlege and Kegan Paul 1986

Finding your Feet, Mary C Lambert, M & J Lambert 1988

Hand and Foot Reflexology, Kevin and Barbara Kunz, Thorsons 1986

Reflexology To-day, Doreen Bayly, Thorsons

Ultrasound Therapy, R Hoogland, B V Enraf-Nonius Delft 1986

The Mastery of Movement, R Laban, Northcote House 1980

Way of Harmony: A guide to the Soft Martial Arts, Howard Reid, Unwin Hyman 1985

Alternative Health: Alexander Technique, Chris Stevens, Optima 1987

Book of Yoga, Sivanananda Yoga Centre, Ebury Press 1987

The Complete Yoga Book, James Hewitt, Rider Books 1983

Relax with Yoga, A Liebers, Oak Tree Press 1960

Yoga Self-Taught, Andre van Lysebeth, Harper 1972

Yoga: Step by Step, Cheryl Isaacson, Thorsons 1986

Creative Visualization, Shakti Gawain, New World Library 1978

Relieve Tension the Autogenic Way, H Lindemann, Abelard-Schulman 1973

Hypnosis and Hypnotherapy: A Patient's Guide, Hellmut WA Karle, BA, APBsS, Thorsons 1988

Inner Conscious Relaxation, Eddie Shapiro, Element Books Limited 1990

Self-Hypnosis and Other Mind-Expanding Techniques, Charles Tebbetts, Martin Breese Publishing 1990

Biofeedback, M Karlins & LM Andrews, Abacus 1979

BIBLIOGRAPHY

Nultritional Medicine, Dr Stephen Davies & Dr Alan Stewart, Pan Books 1987

Holistic Herbal Way to Successful Stress Control, D Hoffman, Thorsons 1986

The Science of Homoeopathy, G Vithoulkas, Thorsons 1986

Bach Flower Therapy, Mechthild Scheffer, Thorsons 1989

Colour Therapy, Mary Anderson, The Aquarian Press 1990

Colours and Numbers 1991, Louise L Hay, Hay House Inc 1991

Healing Power of Colour, Betty Wood, The Aquarian Press 1984

Understanding the Chakras, Peter Rendel, The Aquarian Press 1979

Healing with Crystals and Gems, Daya Sarai Chocron, Samuel Weiser Inc 1983

Healing Music, Andrew Watson & Nevill Drury, Prism Press 1987

Music Therapy, J Alvin, Hutchinson 1985

Sound Medicine: Healing with Music, Voice & Song, Leah Maggie Garfield, Celestial Arts 1987

Alternative Health: Acupuncture, Dr Michael Nightingale, Optima 1987

Alternative Medicine, R Eagle, BBC 1980

Alternative Medicine: A Guide to Natural Therapies, Dr Andrew Stanway, Penguin Books 1986

Alternatives to Drugs: A handbook to health without hazards, Arabella Melville and Colin Johnson, Fontana Paperbacks 1987

Bodypower, Dr Vernon Coleman, Corgi Books 1988

The Chinese Art of Healing, S Palos, Bantam Books, 1971

Dr Vernon Coleman's Guide to Alternative Medicine, Dr Vernon Coleman, Corgi Books 1988

Good Housekeeping Family Health Encyclopaedia, Ebury Press 1989

The Handbook of Complementary Medicine, Stephen Fulder, Coronet Books 1988

The Healer's Hand Book, Georgina Regan and Debbie Shapiro, Element Books 1988

Holistic First Aid: A Handbook for the Home, Dr Michael Nightingale, Optima 1988

Holistic London, Kate Brady and Mike Considine, Brainwave 1990

José Silva: The Man Who Tapped the Secrets of the Human Mind and the Methods He Used, Robert B Stone, PhD, HJ, Kramer Inc 1990

The Medicine Men: A Guide to Natural Medicine, John Lloyd Fraser, Thames/Methuen 1981

Natural Hormone Health: Drug-free ways to manage your life, Arabella Melville, Thorsons 1990

Osteopathic Self-Treatment, Leon Chaitow, DO, MRO, Thorsons 1990

The Resurrection of the Body, FM Alexander, Dell 1971

Rudolf Steiner and Holistic Medicine, Francis X King, Rider & Co Ltd 1986

The Taoist Way of Healing, Chee Soo, Aquarian Press 1986

INDEX

acupressure, **84–5**
adrenalin (epinephrine), **9**
air ionization therapy, **94–5**
alcohol intake, **131**
   drinking problems, **48–9**
Alexander, F M, **102**
Alexander technique, **102–7**
allergies to food, **132–3**
anger, **50–1**
anthroposophical medicine, **147**
anxiety
   anxiety attacks, **60**
   treatment approaches for, **44–5, 52–3**
aromas, in smell therapy, **82–3**
aromatherapy, **80–1**
art therapy, **150–1**
asthma, self-hypnosis for, **126**
auto-hypnosis, **126–8**
   autosuggestion and, **120**
   meditation and, **118**
autogenic therapy, **121**
autonomic nervous system, **8–9**
   biofeedback and, **129**
autosuggestion, **120**
Ayurdevic treatment, **72**

Bach, Edward, **141**
Bach flower remedies, **141**
backache
   treatment approaches for, **38–9**
   yoga for, **114–15**

basic relaxation techniques, **55–69**
   muscle relaxation, **56–9**
bathing, **92**
Bayly, Doreen, **86**
Benjamin, Harry, **134**
biofeedback, **129**
blind people, colour recognition by, **143**
blood pressure, herbal remedies for hypertension, **137**
Bovis, Antoine, **152**
breathing techniques
   basic techniques, **60–3**
   breath meditation, **118**
   colour breathing, **145**
   healing breath, **62**
   sun and moon breath, **63**
breathlessness, **42–3**
bubble meditation, **119**
burns, negative ion therapy for, **95**
Burns, Robert, **91**

caffeine, **130, 131**
chakras, **143, 145**
   in gem therapy, **146**
clinical ecology (nutritional medicine), **130–3**
clothing, colours of, **145**
colic, aromatherapy for, **81**
colitis
   diet-related, **135**
   herbal remedies for, **137**
colour therapy, **142–5**
   crystal/gem therapy, **146**

constipation, **40–1**
cortisol, **9**
Coué, Emile, **120**
Couéism, **120**
cramp, **38–9**
crystal therapy, **146**

dance therapy, **147**
depression
   aromatherapy for, **81**
   herbal remedies for, **137**
   homoeopathic remedy for, **139**
   negative ion therapy for, **95**
   treatment approaches for, **52–3**
diarrhoea
   aromatherapy for, **81**
   herbal remedies for, **137**
   homoeopathic remedy for, **139**
   treatment approaches for, **40–1**
diet
   cleansing diets, **134**
   nutritional medicine, **130–3**
   over-eating, **48–9**
digestive problems
   aromatherapy for, **81**
   autogenic therapy for, **121**
   treatment approaches for, **40–1**
Do-In, **84**
drawing, **150–1**
drinking problems, **48–9**
Duncan, Isadora, **147**

eating problems
   nutritional medicine and, **130–3**
   over-eating, **48–9**
eczema, **95**
electrical stimulation, in TENS therapy, **96**
endorphins, **9, 96**
   released during dancing, **147**
   released during toning, **149**
epinephrine (adrenalin), **9**
Epsom salts, **92**
essential oils, **80–1**
eurhythmy, **147**
evening primrose oil, **137**
exercise, to reduce stress, **14**

facial massage, **74–5**
faith healing, **124–5**
fasting, **135**
fatigue, **46–7**
   yoga for, **116–17**
Federation of American Spiritual Healers, **124**
Feldenkrais method, **108–9**
Feldenkrais, Moshe, **108**
"fight or flight" response, **8–9**
Fitzgerald, William, **86**
floatation tanks, **92**
flowers
   Bach flower remedies, **141**
   in smell therapy, **83**
food
   allergies/intolerance, **40, 132–3**

INDEX

nutritional medicine, **130–3**
over-eating, **48–9**

Gattefossé, **80**
gem therapy, **146**
Ghadiali, Dinshah, **142**
Golden Ratio/Golden Section, **153**

Hahnemann, C, **138**
headaches
  aromatherapy for, **81**
  autogenic therapy for, **121**
  diet-related, **135**
  due to caffeine withdrawal, **131**
  herbal remedies for, **137**
  homoeopathic remedy for, **139**
  negative ion therapy for, **95**
  treatment approaches for, **38–9**
healers and healing, **124–5**
healing breath, **62**
herbalism, **136–7**
Hering, Constantine, **140**
homoeopathy, **138–41**
hydrotherapy, **90–3**
hypertension, herbal remedies for, **137**
hyperventilation, **60**
hypnotherapy, **126–8**
  see also self-hypnosis

indigestion
  aromatherapy for, **81**
  herbal remedies for, **137**
  homoeopathic remedy for, **139**

treatment approaches for, **40–1**
Ingham, Eunice, **86**
inhalation
  in aromatherapy, **80–1**
  in herbalism, **136**, **137**
insomnia
  aromatherapy for, **81**
  diet-related, **135**
  herbal remedies for, **137**
  homoeopathic remedy for, **139**
  self-hypnosis for, **126**
  treatment approaches for, **46–7**
ionizers, **94–5**
irritable bowel syndrome see colitis

jacuzzis, **91**
juice diet, **134**

Kent, James, **140**
Kirlian photography, **143**
Kneipp, Father Sebastian, **90–1**

"laying on of hands", **124**
libido, loss of, **48–9**
life events, stress and, **10**
lifestyles, stressful, **16–35**
Ling, Per Henrik, **72**
lung problems, **95**

mantra meditation, **119**
massage, **72–9**
  aromatherapy and, **80–1**
  foot massage aids, **89**
  quick massage, **75**

self-massage, **78–9**
techniques, **72–3**
meditation, **118–19**
Mesmer, Franz Anton, **126**
metamorphic therapy, **89**
migraine
  diet related, **132**, **135**
  herbal remedies for, **137**
  homoeopathic remedy for, **139**
  self-hypnosis for, **126**
muscle aches/pains
  aromatherapy for, **81**
  homoeopathic remedy for, **139**
  sound therapy for, **97**
  swimming for, **93**
  treatment approaches for, **38–9**
muscle relaxation
  basic technique, **56–9**
  warming-up/stretching exercises, **66–9**
muscle twitching, **42–3**
music therapy, **148–9**

naturopathy, **134–5**
nausea, **40–1**
negative ion therapy, **94–5**
nervous system, autonomic, **8–9**, **129**
nutritional medicine, **130–3**

obsessive behaviour, **50–1**
oils
  essential oils, **80–1**
  evening primrose oil, **137**
  for facial massage, **74**

pain relief
  gate-control theory of, **96**, **84**
  massage for, **73**
  natural hormones and, **96**
  sound therapy for, **97**
  swimming for, **93**
  TENS therapy for, **96**
  treatment approaches for, **38–9**
painting, **150–1**
palpitations, **42–3**
panic attacks, **60**
pattern therapy, **152–3**
perfumes, **82**, **83**
personal relaxation programmes, **15–35**
physiotherapy, **73**
  ultrasound therapy in, **97**
placebos, **122**
plants
  Bach flower remedies, **141**
  herbalism, **136–7**
  in smell therapy, **83**
posture, **64–5**
  Alexander technique and, **102–7**
  common faults of, **102–7**
pre-menstrual tension, **44–5**
Priessnitz, Vincent, **90**
pyramid therapy, **152–3**

reflexology, **86–9**
  metamorphic technique, **89**
relaxometer, **129**
Rescue Remedy (of Bach), **141**
respiratory disorders, **95**

157

INDEX

retirement
  planning ahead for, **15**
  stresses of, **32**

St John, Robert, **89**
saunas, **92**
scents, in smell therapy, **82–3**
Schults, Johannes, **121**
self-healing, **124–5**
self-hypnosis, **126–8**
  autosuggestion and, **120**
  meditation and, **118**
self-massage, **78–9**
sex
  casual sex, **48–9**
  loss of libido, **48–9**
  to relieve tension, **14**

shiatsu, **84–5**
sitz bath, **92**
sleep problems, **46–7**
smell therapy, **82–3**
  aromatherapy, **80–1**
smoking, **48–9**
sound therapy, **97**
  music therapy, **148–9**
  toning therapy, **149**
spas, **90**, **91**
spiritual healing, **124–5**
Steiner, Rudolf, **147**
stress, **7–13**
  life events and, **10**
  signs and symptoms of, **11–13**
  stressful lifestyles, **16–35**

stretching exercises, **66–9**
sun and moon breath, **63**
swimming, **91**, **93**

T'ai chi chuan (T'ai chi), **98–101**
TENS therapy, **96**
tiredness, **46–7**
  yoga for, **116–17**
toning therapy, **149**
transcendental meditation, **118**, **119**
transcutaneous electrical nerve stimulation, **96**
trataka meditation, **119**
Turkish baths, **92**
twitching, **42–3**

ulcers
  diet-related, **135**
  treatment approaches for, **40–1**
ultrasound, **97**

visualization therapy, **122–3**

warming-up exercises, **66–9**
worry *see* anxiety

yin and yang, **101**
yoga, **110–17**

zazen meditation, **118**
zone therapy, **86**

INDEX

The Publishers would like to thank the following individuals for their help with particular sections of this book:

MASSAGE AND T'AI CHI CHUAN
Susan Mumford of The Bennet & Luck Natural Health Centre, 54 Islington Park Street, Islington, London N1 1PX

ALEXANDER TECHNIQUE
Stephen Cooper of The Bloomsbury Alexander Centre, Bristol House, 80a Southampton Row, Bloomsbury, London, WC1.

FELDENKRAIS METHOD
Garet Newell of Somatics, PO Box 1207, Hove, East Sussex, BN3 2GG.

YOGA
Mira Mehta of The Iyengar Yoga Institute, 223a Randolph Avenue, London W9 1NL, and the yoga teachers who performed the poses illustrated in the book – Jackie Langdon, Bill Rowles, Judith Smith and Ian Tittley.

The Publishers would also like to thank the models Mandy Wood, David Kemp and Bruce Low; Penny Gibbons at Grayshott Hall, Grayshott, near Hindhead, Surrey, who supplied the two photographs in the Hydrotherapy section; and Wholistic and Life Extension, 290 Hanworth Road, Hampton, Middlesex, GU12 3EP, for lending the pictures as reference for the illustrations in the Colour Therapy and the Crystal and Gem Therapy sections.